NATURAL HERBAL THERAPY

A SCRIPTURAL, TORAH BASED WAY TO RECLAIM YOUR HEALTH NATURALLY

LUCINDA GIBBS ROBINSON

Other books by Lucinda Gibbs Robinson-

SHOT DETOX

And others on www.amazon.com

TABLE OF CONTENTS

Dedication

This book is dedicated to my Dad, Thomas Maxwell Gibbs, Jr. who first told me about the Creator(Yehovah, Yehowah, Yahweh), "Jesus" (Yehoshua, Yehshua) and the real Scriptures. After he read the whole Scriptures for the first time, he would not touch unclean animals for food again. He said when he stopped eating the unclean animals his anger left him. He loved natural foods and thought it was very important to eat right, be moderate in your eating, exercise (he walked in the woods at all times of the year watching wild game), and that how you treated people affected the Creator's blessings on you. He caught scores of salmon from Lake Michigan near Manistee, Michigan and gave them away to poor people in the area. He took us as children to the Finger Lakes in New York State to pick delicious apples, peaches, nectarines, apricots, red raspberries, black raspberries, cherries, strawberries, and, of course, grapes. Those memories are so sweet and precious to me. He hunted pheasant and turkeys. He and his brothers always had a great, friendly competition going on whether it was in fishing or hunting. They were always there the first day of trout fishing season at the locally famous Catherine Creek where the men stood sometimes shoulder-to-shoulder fishing for those beautiful trout. He hunted deer every year and knew well ahead of time where the deer and turkey were by his walks in the woods. He read extensively at times on natural treatments for disease and tried many remedies on himself. His treats were fresh fruit. He was always happy and healthy. I cannot remember one day when he was "down". Everyone he met was an instant friend and the conversation always eventually came to the Creator, His Son, and the Written Word in the friendliest way. He talked easily, freely, and earnestly about his blessings and experiences of the Father in heaven's intervention in his life to others in the hopes of convincing them to" "taste and see that the Creator is good". Although he was the middle child of his family, he outlived all his brothers and sisters. When he died at 86, he was on NO prescription medicine and died peacefully in his sleep after a joy filled day of attending his

8

granddaughter's (my daughter's) wedding. His memory, his encouragement, his happy and hopeful attitude, his love of truth will always be with me until the day I....

CREDITS

Thanks, CREDIT, and More Credit

I would like to thank the following people for their help in this endeavor--

My big sister Beverly who said she knew I could do it when I did not think I could.

My husband, David, who, YEARS AGO, bought me a computer, "So you can write your book". I did!

My oldest son, Wesley, who told me to get busy on the book when the last and youngest of his 7 siblings, Jerusha, left our home for nursing school at UNC Chapel Hill and who gave me unlimited computer and publication help. I can not thank him enough for his constant, eager, patient, and cheerful help to me.

Edaphanie Pettigrew, RN, for all the times she fixed herbs for the sick in our church and her dedication to natural treatments.

All my detractors who have called me the "witch doctor" and the "parasite lady" and the "colon cleanse freak" and the "winkiologist", "crazy" and "just plain wrong", who only gave me more energy to get the real truth out about natural health and herbal treatments. Bless your hearts.

All my clients who have been appreciative of the effort I poured into each one as they would let me.

All my AIDS and cancer clients who clung to hope, took their health future into their own hands, and WON!

And lastly, but ever first in my heart, the great Creator in Heaven Who inspired me and gave me wisdom and directed me to knowledge and encouraged my heart along the way through His spirit and saints. Use this, now, O Father, to help throngs get well!

I started this book in 1996. It is 2011 today. I worked on and off on it from time to time. But nearly every day during that time there were daily urgings in my inner most being to finish the book. I had completely stopped in early 2010 for awhile. One night I had a dream.

I saw a large primitive clinic seemingly in Africa. There were many simple beds with very sick and weak people in them. At the foot of each bed, there was a person in pure white clothing. All in the beds and at the foot of the beds where looking at me and imploring me with their very sad eyes to help them. I awoke and was so sad, but I knew the meaning the moment I woke up. The information the Creator of Heaven had so graciously allowed me to see and see work would help those people, and they needed it now.

BOOKS YOU SHOULD READ

My book is partly a culmination of many authors', researchers', other books' information and inspiration. As in all scientific study, one fact builds upon another. One researcher's discoveries are founded on the platform of previous researcher's findings. Each of the following books contains so much valuable information you need to know TODAY, I urge you to read some these wonderful books to broaden your personal horizons in this wonderful field of health, natural health, herbs, and what affects your health. What I will tell you in this book will be built on what has already been discovered in these books. AND THIS IS JUST A START....

BACK TO EDEN

CHANGE YOUR BRAIN, CHANGE YOUR BODY

SILENT SPRING

HEALING WITHOUT MEDICATION

MAD COWBOY

NO MORE BULL

DIET FOR A SMALL PLANET

DIET FOR A NEW AMERICA

LET'S EAT RIGHT TO KEEP FIT

LET'S HAVE HEALTHY CHILDREN

LET'S GET WELL

NONE OF THESE DISEASES

IT'S ALL IN YOUR HEAD

THE ENCYCLOPEDIA OF HEALTH AND NUTRITION

THE HALLELUYAH DIET

THE CURE FOR ALL DISEASES

PERSCRIPTION FOR NATURAL CURES

PERSCRIPTION FOR NUTRITIONAL HEALING

PERSCRIPTION FOR HERBAL HEALING

THE SCRIPTURES

COMPLETE JEWISH BIBLE

HEALING OILS OF THE BIBLE

THE SCRIPTURES

AND MANY, MANY MORE

INTRODUCTION

We do not have a health CARE crisis in our country. There are plenty of places to get conventional treatments for poor health. And for free! in many desperate cases. We are having, however, an HEALTH crisis and that crisis is caused by a REAL FOOD crisis and a CHEMICAL crisis in our country.

It is not that there is not enough food or not enough varieties of food. We are blessed to have so many varieties of food from scores of countries available in our neighborhood stores. It is that the food we have so abundantly available to us is contaminated by herbicides, pesticides, food additives, preservatives, artificial food colorings, artificial flavorings, and additives of all kinds. Add to these the hundreds of NON-FOOD chemicals that are touching our foods in growing it, processing it, and preserving it. Now add to this all the conventional drugs, over the counter drugs, immunizations, vaccinations, innoculations, flu shots, and recreational drugs taken so frequently by so many. Now add the variable contents of well and municipal water sources. And to that add the chemicals in our air from chemtrails and home environments. Most of these chemicals were never intended to enter the human body. Is it any wonder our bodies are not "well"? To me, it is amazing we are as well as we are!

We are VERY chemically toxic. We are so chemically TOXIC that the normal functions of our bodies can not proceed normally as bodies used to be able to function.

We have ceased to eat REAL FOOD! How did this ever happen and when? Organically grown, whole foods are THE ONLY REAL FOODS. Up until about 60 years ago, it was the ONLY food available. How much of it have you had TODAY? YESTERDAY? THE LAST WEEK? THE LAST YEAR?

If you are a believer in the One Great Creator (YEHOVAH,YEHOWAY,YAHUAH,YAHWAY,ETC.), then you believe the earth is approximately 6,000 years old. For approximately 5,850 of those years, people only used and had available to them all natural medicinal cures such as organically grown foods, herbs, water, sunshine, mineral baths, heat, cold, fresh air, rest, fasting, natural based skin ointments made of natural oils and natural elements, etc. Those who studied and used these avenues regularly generally lived long and healthy lives.

They worked long and hard hours in sunshine and cold, year in and year out. For most, their very IMMEDIATE future existence (if they wanted to be alive NEXT YEAR) depended on how hard they worked TODAY to grow and preserve food.

These people ONLY had available to them organically grown food. The soil was replenished every year with the valuable nutrients they had eaten in the food harvested from that soil though vegetable and animal manure. This formed a perfect recycling pattern. Not much was lost from the soil year to year.

Through generations and by experience, people passed down the knowledge of what field grown herbs were good for what ailment. Most of the herbs gathered were grown in virgin soil. These herbs were absolutely jam packed with nutrients.

The essential oils from the plants were extracted and used as barter for other goods because of their great value and encompassing uses.

The water, also, was pure from springs and creeks and rivers. There was nothing there to pollute their pureness! Most living, moving waters pulled valuable nutrients along their moving courses and deposited them along the shores and banks for human use.

These people spent hours upon hours, working hard every muscle in bodies, in the sunshine, usually in modest, natural fiber clothing that allowed only a moderate amount of sunshine to actually shine on their skins and keeping their body temperatures nearly constant. This hard work kept muscles moving, keeping bones strong, posture straight, and digestion working well.

They breathed in huge amounts of fresh air as they worked hard, and the primitive construction of their all-natural material homes allowed fresh air in even in the times when they had to be indoors.

Their diet was mostly easily stored root vegetables, dried berries, and dried green vegetables with some grains and very infrequent meat consumption. It was hard work to go find meat and, once an animal was killed, it had to be eaten within 12 to 24 hours before it spoiled or it had to be dried or smoked immediately. To have meat was usually at a special festival or just weekly, according to the family's strength and means. The few domesticated animals they killed were allowed to roam freely nearby to eat what they desired before they were killed and each had little contact with other animals.

The food they ate was very nutritious. It was grown in virgin soil, many times gathered in the wild. It had the maximum amount of nutrients its genetics would allow unhindered by any foreign chemicals, being grown in organic soil. They did not feel hungry or have as many cravings as frequently as we do because of the food's high nutritional content.

Most of these people were accustomed to NOT having 3 meals a day, and certainly no snacks. It was no hardship or time of panic if they did not eat that regularly. They ate when hungry or only 1 or 2 times a day at the most. Or they ate sufficiently when the food was plentiful and rested from eating when there was little or none. If they followed the Scriptural pattern, they had two week long festivals (Passover or Unleavened Bread in the spring and Sukkoth or Feast of Tabernacles in the fall) 6 months apart where any food was freely consumed to their heart's delight near in time following two very intense work periods of harvesting.

After all the work they did, they rested well, usually retiring near sunset and arising before sunrise, giving them 7 to 8 hours to rest in the summer and 8 to 9 hours in the winter. The last light they saw was the restful dark blue of the sky. Well over half of that sleeping time was before midnight. If they followed the Scriptural pattern, every seventh day, they completely rested from any physical and material labor and concentrated on adding to their spiritual knowledge.

They lived in generational homes, groups, and dwellings where older members of the family lived with or near and helped the younger married family members with cooking, caring for the "grands", and passing down and teaching good, proven advice on may subjects pertaining to family living.

The groups who followed the SCRIPTURAL COMMANDS buried their human waste (Deuteronomy 23:13) and washed themselves and their belongings frequently (Leviticus 13-17).

They quarantined sick people (Leviticus 14).

They lived in separate buildings or areas from ANY of their animals.

They never ate scavenger or predator ("unclean" or non-kosher) animals (Leviticus 11 and Deuteronomy 14). They even refrained from touching the dead carcasses of these unclean animals (Leviticus 11:8).

They limited themselves to one virgin sexual partner for life (Leviticus 21:14).

They completely burned or dismantled any home or belonging that had strange growths of mold or fungus in them (Leviticus 14:40-45).

They wore natural fiber clothing (linen and wool). All of their belongings and household furnishings and fabrics in the living space were of natural fiber and product (wood, leather,metal) origin.

They used water and fire to disinfect belongings taken as booty or used items from other family groups (Numbers 31:23).

When they needed medicine, they turned to medicinal herbs which had high concentrations of valuable healing chemicals. They understood the anti-viral, anti-bacterial, anti-fungal, and anti-parasitic properties of herbs, such as myrrh, garlic, figs, onions, cucumbers, and hyssop (Psalms 104:14).

They extracted the potent essential oils from their local plants to use as medicine and for barter.

AH, it all seemed so perfect then—or was it?

People got sick. Some children died really early because of improper sanitation, getting chilled in drafty homes and sitting in wet clothes during potty training or from just crawling on dirt floors. Sometimes a worn out new mother just could not produce enough milk for her baby because so much of her energy was being used to just to keep up all the work she was required to do each day. Childhood respiratory ailments were hard to cure when children were playing in dirt all the time or living in draughty or smoke filled homes.

If you broke a bone or had a large open wound from an accident, it was almost always a death sentence. It was very difficult to keep a large open area of skin meticulously clean. If a tooth was infected or broken off, the pain could last for years and the infection from it might eventually kill you.

Women died at childbirth very frequently because of infection or unstopped blood loss.

Although natural cures could have helped all of these things, the KNOWLEDGE of those cures and remedies was not available to EVERYONE, or the resources to procure those helps. Many years and many discoveries have happened since more primitive days, but there are STILL societies on this earth RIGHT NOW that suffer from all the above problems.

In spite of all of man's progress, there also still are areas where there is gross ignorance on the value of natural cures in even developed cultures.

Every book I have ever read on the subject of the use of herbs and natural treatments versus the use of conventional drugs so thoroughly states the harmful effects of a few unwisely used herbs without telling the wonderful effects of the hundreds of powerful and harmless herbs that it scares and discourages any reader to want to even try using herbs for treatment. That is why I, after 37 years as an herbalist and believer, am writing this book. There have already been written many books by faith-oriented authors on the subject of natural health. Why other one? This one is from the perspective of Scriptural principles, real organic food, and POWERFUL, BUT GENTLE HERBS being the main factor in natural healing – a subject I have not seen anyone be bold enough, or maybe experienced enough, to write about with confidence.

It also is a book to encourage those who have very serious diseases. These are the ones in chronic or critical condition. I am talking about the ones where the doctor says there are only a few weeks or days left. Following a natural lifestyle will bring about healing. But if death is approaching fast, the knowledge given in THIS BOOK OF THE USES OF HERBS TO SPEED HEALING will be a literal lifesaver for many. My interaction with hundreds of people over the years has shown such excellent results.

Many of the Scriptural based books already existing tell of a Creator prescribed lifestyle to recovery health. These books show a lifestyle that takes a year or two to fully recover health. But THIS book gives information on concentrated herbal formulas and regimens that will help the person who only has A FEW WEEKS TO LIVE TO TOTALLY RECOVER very quickly before their time runs out. It is a fast track to health adding to already known healing factors using already proven methods.

In 1971, while a child development/nutrition/consumer advocacy/ communications student at Cornell University, someone gave me a book telling of Dr. John Harvey Kellogg's Battle Creek Sanitarium. It was a 1,000 bed health spa, as we would call it today, where the rich, famous, educated, exhausted, and very ill people of his time would come to recover of all their various ills. He used organic, natural, whole foods, water treatments, sunshine, exercise, spiritual study and prayer, controlled fasting, herbs, freshly prepared juices, rest, fresh air, music, and garden viewing to heal, and it worked! I wondered-why are not we employing this same method now? When as a new believer in Messiah and the Scriptures, I saw this was a perfect way to help people while pointing them to other Scriptural approved ways of superior living.

Thus started my 40 plus year study of natural treatments for disease, with a concentration on the use of herbs, and the naturally formed chemicals in those herbs, for healing. I always had as my criteria for learning about and incorporating any treatment the question—Is this treatment consistent with the principles of the Scriptures? Is there anything in this treatment that would conflict with Scriptural teachings?

As a wedding gift in 1973, Bro. Robert Baker of Brooklyn, NY gave my husband, David, and me a book named BACK TO EDEN by Jethro Kloss. This book microscoped my attention on a subject I was totally hoping to find out more about. While rearing 8 children (including 6 home births with one being twins!), I continued studying all I could on this subject matter. In this time period, I home schooled our 8 children for 14 years. One year, I taught 5 different grades while breastfeeding twins!! I still read as much as I could on the subject. At times it was only in the bathroom behind a locked door while I accomplished other things at the same time!

People I knew knew my passion for this subject and starting asking me what I had found out about certain ailments. Soon I had developed my own regimens for different conditions. I told my first "clients" that what I have found might not work specifically for them, but that we could try. Over time, I continued to work out regimens that worked consistently in most doctor-diagnosed conditions. As time passed, many people said you have to write all this down in a book so that others can benefit from it farther than your own locality and your own mortality.

With the advent of the Internet, I could research in more books and studies and researches and journals than anyone could ever possibly personally own. Now, because of the Internet, I had available studies from South American universities, and those in India, Germany, Switzerland, and many others. I could learn of one researcher's small finding and add it to another researcher's small finding. In time, I compiled many useful treatments and/or combined specific supplements that had cured a few or many people of a specific health problem. Adding this to what was already known made the regimen I suggested to my clients have a higher probability of helping them. And it did!

Now it can be said after hundreds of clients, locally and around the world by appointment, letters, Internet, and phone, I am well satisfied I chose to follow my passion. In high school, I was asked what I wanted to do in life, I remember saying, "Something to help people." I feel I have been a bystander of miracles, watching clients who have given up on the doctors, or whom the doctors have said to go home and die, get well and live many more productive years. And most of those people continue, alive today, and are among my best friends!

I am especially grateful for the results of my AIDS and cancer regimens. Most have been cancer free in 6 to 12 weeks on my cancer regimen. And some have been "virus undetectable" in as short a time as 4 weeks on my AIDS regimen.

My first working with an AIDS patient came in 1996. A friend of mine had a brother with AIDS. She asked me if I thought I could help him. I told her I had not yet worked with anyone with AIDS, but I had already formulated in my mind after much study how I would treat an AIDS patient with herbs and other natural agents if asked. He started the regimen I designed for him. In four weeks he had a medical appointment and another HIV test. He tested "virus undetectable". His story was quite interesting from a human standpoint as his sister had several churches praying for him as he took the treatment. MANY OTHER CLIENTS AFTER THAT UNTIL NOW HAVE TAKEN THE SAME TREATMENT AND HAVE HEALED THEMSELVES.

The basis of these regimens entails getting rid of parasites and toxic chemicals and restoring function in every area of his body by using high powered, but gentle, herbs.

I am happy to say that it does not matter how bad the disease, if you have the right medicine. And there is a natural medicine or medicines and help out there for any sickness man can contract, in spite of what any doctor tells you. Just because the medical doctors do not KNOW of a cure does not mean it does not exist. Conventional medicine or allopathic medicine doctors can only doctor their patients to the extent of their own knowledge and to the extent their individual medical schools have taught them. And most medical schools are severely lacking in natural and herbal medicinal knowledge AND WHAT THEY HAVE BEEN TAUGHT. Conventional medical schools are sending doctors out to treat patients without fully equipping the medical students with ALL the knowledge they will need to HEAL and CURE fully and especially in the herbal and natural treatment areas. I hope this book will fill in the gaps, to a small degree, that believers, and even some doctors, are looking for. I feel every medical doctor should have at least 2 years of herbal and natural treatment schooling before being able to PRACTICE!

Most of the people who have contacted me over the years for help at my counseling service named Natural Herbal Therapy fall mainly into 5 categories.

The first group is Christian believers, Messianic believers, or Jewish believers who have decided to follow the Scriptures and have decided to use no conventional medicine at all no matter what the outcome. They feel it is morally and Scripturally wrong to use anything in their bodies that will harm it in any way. If they die, they have decided, it is the Creator's will, as they will not take any harmful substance into their bodies.

The second group is people who have been to the doctor and tried all the treatments that conventional medicine can offer and they are no better (and usually worse because of the side effects of the treatments AND THE COMPOUNDED EFFECTS OF MULTIPLE DRUGS!). These realize that conventional treatments are not helping them get better, so they have given up on the doctors and want to try something else.

The third group is clients who have been told by the doctor to go home and die. So they feel they have nothing to lose by trying a one last chance ANYTHING to save their lives.

The fourth group is those who have just gotten a diagnosis and want to try natural treatments first before even considering conventional treatments.

The fifth group is those who have studied natural treatments and have quite a bit of knowledge in the natural treatment area. But they just have not come upon the particular combinations that will specifically help them. They just need a little direction and fine tuning to complete their healing.

Everyone in all five groups comes with a doctor's diagnosis in hand.

I am a believer in the supreme Father in Heaven and His great mercies to us mere humans. I meet a lot of believers who feel they do not have all the information they need in physical and spiritual issues. These believers are growing up. They want more and more complete information on how to have faith in and obey the Creator more completely. Their vision is clearing and focusing more on the direct commands of the Creator in His word. They want to experience the fullness of the Creator's blessings He has for them. They are weary of being deceived and led astray in every area of life. They are tired of impotent half-truths. They are tired, spiritually and physically, of being dragged around with no results. They are awakening to the benefits here and into eternity of doing EVERYTHING the Creator's way. My desire is that I might add truthful, useful information in just my one niche of study, health and natural and herbal therapy, that can vastly improve the quality and length of the lives of anyone, but especially those dedicated to serving the Creator they may live longer and stronger and that through their work many more may be brought to the Messiah and the laws of right living, the TORAH.

I also hope that others see that the TRUE answers to all of life's troubles are very simple, easy, and quite painless, all in accordance with the Creator's tremendous love, pity, and mercy toward us. He has a perfect, beautiful plan for everyone, and included in this plan is excellent health, simply and easily taken care of. Although we may be torn from the right and true path at times, He is ever willing to show us the way back to LIFE.

All of us have had friends and relatives who have sought health through very painful, debilitating, disfiguring, and further health robbing means. The plans explained here give hope, healing, repair, restoration, strength, and energy from the onset of starting them, using only things the Creator set here at creation. May the unbeliever be awakened to the love of the Creator by these facts alone.

This book is about my personal experience as an herbalist and the things I have seen work in very specific conditions in the 40 years I have been helping people.

For the reader, this book picks up where THE MAKERS DIET, THE HALLELUYAH DIET, MAD COWBOY, THE CHINA STUDY, DIET FOR A SMALL PLANET, LET'S EAT RIGHT TO KEEP FIT, and DIET FOR A NEW AMERICA and others stop. It gives you very specific information to overcome very specific, critical, and chronic health problems. It uses the principles of the Scriptures and takes it many steps deeper. It shows you how to speed up your healing if you need help very fast. It gives ways to help even the weakest person.

There are also principles shown in this book that will help almost any problem or even if you are not sure exactly what your problem is.

This book is also written in the simplest of language so a child may read it and may help himself, his parents, or his grandparents get better from a severe illness.

I HOPE MY ADVICE TO YOU WILL BE TAKEN AS A LOVING MOTHER, GRANDMOTHER, OR LOVING FRIEND SHOWING YOU COMMON SENSE AND FREEING KNOWLEDGE AND WISDOM.

In all of this, I gently offer the information you need to HELP YOURSELF. It is possible to have great health; I want to show you how.

I am a Messianic/Hebrew roots/ Scripturalist believer. Because of this, I will use the word Creator (Yahweh, Yah, Yehovah, Yehowah, the name of the one true "god" (elohim) in heaven who created all things), and the word Messiah (Yahushuah, Yehoshua, Yehshua, Y'Shua, Joshua, "Jesus") for the Son He gave to die for our sins throughout this book. I will call the written word of the Creator, the Scriptures.

CHAPTER ONE

IT IS THE CREATOR'S WILL WE BE IN GOOD HEALTH.

This may seem like a funny statement to start out a book on sickness. But there are many people who think it is the Creator's will we all have various types of diseases from time to time. If not, why do they accept a lower level of health? Why do they think it is perfectly normal or the will of the Creator that 1 out of 4 of their friends is going to die of cancer? Why do they think it is acceptable that one in five of their friends will die of a heart attack? They have to believe it is somehow the Creator's will to be sick and eventually decline in health. They believe somehow, someway the Creator has a plan for all of this.

Christian believers have the same proportions of degenerative health problems in the total population right now that the unbelievers have. Does that not stir you? It is much more than just BELIEVING that sends good health to you.

Think about this. Do you know ANYONE right now who is perfectly healthy? Almost everyone I know over 20 YEARS OLD has SOME degenerative disease symptoms. To me, it is almost enough to drive you mad. How is it that nearly everyone I know is sick or weak in some way? It is rather astounding I think.

And so many are young people who should be at the peak of their health!

And so many children are born with defects of some kind. Right now, we have more defects per thousand births than we have EVER had in the USA! We have more defects per thousand births than countries where a simple, even if monotonous, natural foods diet is the staple!

Compare real photos of Civil War soldiers (who were mostly teenagers) and young people today. In the Civil War pictures, their teeth were naturally straight and large, the faces rounded, nearly perfect complexions, wide open eyes, slim but erect posture. Too many of today's teenagers are thin faced, crooked teeth, decayed teeth, sallow and pimpled complexion, poor postured, and frankly not as full faced beautiful as when only ORGANIC, natural foods were available.

How have we gotten this way? Why is there so much sickness? Is it normal for a spiritual person to be continually sick? Or is it normal for a believer to go from one sickness to the next sickness?

The Scriptural example is just not so. Those who DID THE CREATOR'S COMPLETE WILL lived long lives and had great strength and vitality until their last day. Moses is the prime example. The Creator just took his breath away (Deuteronomy 34:7). He died of old age, as the saying goes. In the Scriptures it just says, "He slept with his fathers" of most of the well known Scriptural figures. Of very few Scriptural characters does it say "he died of an illness". My own Dad lived for 86 years, was on no prescription medicine when he died, had no known sickness, had lots of strength, and an alert mind. He just died in his sleep.

Why do we SOMETIMES attribute to the Creator as His will for all this sickness all around us? The Scripture says if we do ALL His will ALL sickness will be taken away from us (Exodus15:26) It is as if an invisible shield is to be given us against sickness if we do His will.(Deuteronomy 28:21,22) Why are not we expecting and experiencing this today?

Is it that part of doing His will is partly our action in PHYSICAL THINGS THAT GUARD OUR HEALTH? That is what I believe. I believe if we treat our bodies the way the SCRIPTURE shows us, WE ARE FOLLOWING SCIENTIFICALLY SOUND PRINCIPLES that lead us to superior health. From the Scriptural, therefore spiritual physical commands we follow, we receive physical health. Scientific research has proven that everything that is mentioned in the Scripture about health is scientifically bona fide!

Is it also true that because we are not living the same SPIRITUAL LIVES OUR ANCESTORS DID, we are reaping the reward of poor health?

There is no promise in Scripture that if we just eat organic foods, exercise, rest, drink pure water, keep clean, etc. we will have good health! Remember, even in the earthly time of Messiah, this is ALL the people had and He had to heal thousands of them! Health, strength, and protection from disease was promised to those who kept FULL COVENANT with the Creator! The Scriptures address this many times in places such as-

"My son, forget not my law; but let thine heart keep my commandments: For LENGTH OF DAYS, and LONG LIFE, and peace, shall they add to thee. Let not mercy and truth forsake thee: bind them about thy neck; write them upon the table of thine heart: So shalt thou find favour and good understanding in the sight of elohim and the Creator. Trust in the Creator with all thine heart; and lean not unto thine own understanding. In all thy ways acknowledge him, and he shall direct thy paths. Be not wise in thine own eyes: fear the Creator, and depart from evil. It shall be HEALTH to thy navel, and marrow to thy bones." (Proverbs 3:1-8 KJV),

"My son, attend to my words; incline thine ear unto my sayings. Let them not depart from thine eyes; keep them in the midst of thine heart. For they are LIFE unto those that find them, and HEALTH TO ALL THEIR FLESH. Keep thy

HEART with all diligence; for out of it are the issues of LIFE." (Proverbs 4:20-23 KJV),

"There is that speaketh like the piercings of a sword: but the TONGUE OF THE WISE IS HEALTH." (Proverbs 12:18 KJV),

"Cry aloud, spare not, lift up thy voice like a trumpet, and shew my people their transgression, and the house of Jacob their sins. Yet they seek me daily, and delight to know my ways, as a nation that did righteousness, and forsook not the ordinance of their elohim: they ask of me the ordinances of justice; they take delight in approaching to elohim. Wherefore have we fasted, say they, and thou seest not? wherefore have we afflicted our soul, and thou takest no knowledge? Behold, in the day of your fast ye find pleasure, and exact all your labours. Behold, ye fast for strife and debate, and to smite with the fist of wickedness: ye shall not fast as ye do this day, to make your voice to be heard on high. Is it such a fast that I have chosen? a day for a man to afflict his soul? is it to bow down his head as a bulrush, and to spread sackcloth and ashes under him? wilt thou call this a fast, and an acceptable day to the Creator? Is not this the fast that I have chosen? to loose the bands of wickedness, to undo the heavy burdens, and to let the oppressed go free, and that ye break every yoke? Is it not to deal thy bread to the hungry, and that thou bring the poor that are cast out to thy house? when thou seest the naked, that thou cover him; and that thou hide not thyself from thine own flesh? Then shall thy light break forth as the morning, and THINE HEALTH SHALL SPRING FORTH SPEEDILY: and thy righteousness shall go before thee; the glory of the Creator shall be thy rereward. Then shalt thou call, and the Creator shall answer; thou shalt cry, and he shall say, Here I am. If thou take away from the midst of thee the yoke, the putting forth of the finger, and speaking vanity; And if thou draw out thy soul to the hungry, and satisfy the afflicted soul; then shall thy light rise in obscurity, and thy darkness be as the noonday: And the Creator shall guide thee continually, and satisfy thy soul in drought, and make fat thy bones: and thou shalt be like a watered garden, and like a spring of water, whose waters fail not. And they that shall be of thee shall build the old waste places: thou shalt raise up the foundations of many generations; and thou shalt be called, The repairer of the breach, The restorer of paths to dwell in. If thou turn away thy foot from the sabbath, from doing thy pleasure on my holy day; and call the sabbath a delight, the holy of the Creator, honourable; and shalt honour him, not doing thine own ways, nor finding thine own pleasure, nor speaking thine own words: Then shalt thou delight thyself in the Creator, and I will cause thee to ride upon the high places of the earth, and feed thee with the heritage of Jacob thy father: for the mouth of the Creator hath spoken it." (Isaiah 58:1-14 KJV),

"There is NO SOUNDNESS IN MY FLESH BECAUSE OF THINE ANGER; neither is there any rest in my bones because of my sin." (Psalms 38:3 KJV),

"To the chief Musician, A Psalm of David, Blessed is he that considereth the poor: The Creator will deliver him in time of trouble. The Creator will preserve him, and KEEP HIM ALIVE; and he shall be blessed upon the earth: and thou wilt not deliver him unto the will of his enemies. The Creator will STRENGTHEN HIM UPON THE BED OF LANGUISHING: thou wilt MAKE ALL HIS BED IN HIS SICKNESS. I said, the Creator, be merciful unto me: heal my soul; for I have sinned against thee. Mine enemies speak evil of me, When shall he die, and his name perish? And if he come to see me, he speaketh vanity: his heart gathereth iniquity to itself; when he goeth abroad, he telleth it. All that hate me whisper together against me: against me do they devise my hurt. ... Yea, mine own familiar friend, in whom I trusted, which did eat of my bread, hath lifted up his heel against me. But thou, O Creator, be merciful unto me, and raise me up, that I may requite them. By this I know that thou favourest me, because mine enemy doth not triumph over me. And as for me, thou upholdest me in mine integrity, and settest me before thy face for ever. Blessed be the Creator elohim of Israel from everlasting, and to everlasting. Amen, and Amen." (Psalms 41:1-7, 9-13 KJV),

"And the Creator shall smite Egypt: he shall smite and HEAL it: and they shall return even to the Creator, and he shall be intreated of them, and shall HEAL them." (Isaiah 19:22 KJV),

"For this people's heart is waxed gross, and their ears are dull of hearing, and their eyes they have closed; lest at any time they should see with their eyes, and hear with their ears, and should understand with their heart, and should be converted, and I should HEAL them." (Matthew 13:15 KJV),

"He hath blinded their eyes, and hardened their heart; that they should not see with their eyes, nor understand with their heart, and be converted, and I should HEAL them." (John 12:40 KJV) and,

"For the heart of this people is waxed gross, and their ears are dull of hearing, and their eyes have they closed; lest they should see with their eyes, and hear with their ears, and understand with their heart, and should be converted, and I SHOULD HEAL THEM." (Act 28:27 KJV),

as well as many other references. Our Scriptural ancestors loved and feared and practiced the Creator's loving instructions (the Torah) on EVERY aspect of their lives and many believers today have set those beautiful paths of living aside in the supposed name of grace much to their detriment. Messiah saves us, but the TORAH shows us how to live ABOVE the curses of this world and how to attain the blessings in this life-

Deuteronomy 27-30- THESE 4 CHAPTERS REVEAL TO US THE DIVINE WILL OF THE CREATOR! These chapters are clearer than any others in the whole of Scripture as to what EXACTLY the Creator expects of an human being. It reveals how to get the continual intervention of the Creator in your life. He clearly delineates right (righteous) and wrong behaviour and actions. He shows how to be rewarded, protected, prospered, and promoted. He explains why trouble, cursing, waiting, waste, and sickness come into your life. It is all there, plain as the daylight. Exodus 12 through the end of the book of Deuteronomy gives you all the details of this holy, right(eous) lifestyle He blesses!

"And the Creator will TAKE AWAY FROM THEE ALL SICKNESS, and will put NONE OF THESE EVIL DISEASES of Egypt, which thou knowest, upon thee; but will lay them upon all them that hate thee." (Deuteronomy 7:15 KJV),

"Then the Creator will make THY PLAGUES wonderful, and the PLAGUES of thy seed, even great PLAGUES, and of LONG CONTINUANCE, and SORE SICKNESSES, and of long continuance. Moreover he will bring upon thee ALL THE DISEASES of Egypt, which thou wast afraid of; and they shall CLEAVE unto thee. Also EVERY SICKNESS, and EVERY PLAGUE WHICH IS NOT WRITTEN IN THIS BOOK OF THE LAW, them will the Creator bring upon thee, until thou BE DESTROYED." (Deuteronomy 28:59-61 KJV),

"The Creato shall smite thee with a CONSUMPTION, and with a FEVER, and with an INFLAMMATION, and with and EXTREME BURNING, and with the sword, and with blasting, and with mildew; and they shall pursue thee until thou perish." (Deuteronomy 28:22 KJV),

"And the Creator shall separate him unto evil out of all the tribes of Israel, according to all the curses of the covenant that are written in this book of the law:" (Deuteronomy 29:21 KJV),

"And said, If thou wilt diligently hearken to the voice of the Creator your elohim, and wilt do that which is right in his sight, and wilt give ear to his commandments, and keep all his statutes, I will put NONE OF TAHESE DISEASES upon thee, which I have brought upon the Egyptians: for I am the Creator that HEALETH thee." (Exodus 15:26 KJV),

"And ye shall serve the Creator your elohim, and he shall bless thy bread, and thy water; and I will TAKE SICKNESS AWAY from the midst of thee." (Exodus 23:25 KJV),

"Thou shalt keep therefore his statutes, and his commandments, which I command thee this day, that it may GO WELL with thee, and with thy children after thee, and that thou mayest PROLONG THY DAYS upon the earth, which the Creator thy elohim giveth thee, for ever." (Deuteronomy 4:40 KJV), and

"Ye shall walk in all the ways which the Creator your elohim hath commanded you, that ye may LIVE, and that it may BE WELL WITH YOU, and that ye may PROLONG YOUR DAYS in the land which ye shall possess." (Deuteronomy 5:33 KJV).

It is the Creator's grace (divine unmerited influence and favor) that brings us to truth on ANY level or subject. The Torah shows us HOW to live life on the highest plane and with that fullness and abundance Messiah spoke of. He taught the fullness of the laws of the Creator so we could partake of the best and most blessings. The Torah, reaffirmed by Messiah's teachings, shows us how to LIVE!

Dr. Henry W. Wright has studied and observed over years' experience that people who do not live in obedience to the Creator's will and laws can not get rid of their sicknesses until they REPENT. These changes may be forgiving someone, releasing anger, bitterness, and resentment, apologizing to someone for a past fault, or completely changing their behavior and falling back in line with the Words of the Creator in the ways they have erred.

A few people have come to me for hope of healing over the years and once I knew of their spiritual condition, no matter how many natural treatments they had tried, they never got better. In most of these cases, I knew their efforts would be in vain as they had something they needed to get right with the Creator first. Then they would get healed. And they did get healed if they took care of the "Creator offenses". Some others were healed without repenting by the mere grace and mercy of the Creator who most likely just wanted them to know of His love, mercy, and existence. Long suffering as He is, later He would deal with them on those issues.

Besides our not living spiritually as pure as our ancestors, we are also not living in a natural world like people did for the first 5,850 years of history. Man has changed the beautiful, perfect environment the Creator set up from the beginning. We have changed the chemical nature of our foods, water, what we put on our skins, the air we breathe, and what we take into our bodies to make us feel better.

We have stopped eating REAL FOOD! Garden of Eden organic food!

We are ingesting chemicals on our foods, water, medicines, and vaccinations in our flesh that do not belong there nor can be metabolized or broken down as waste.

We do not experience as much natural light as our ancestors did because of indoor electrical lighting and sturdier homes and workplaces and our not having to work the soil for our food.

We do not breathe in as much pure air because of spending too much time indoors in tightly built homes and the pollution of our air from manmade materials of the THINGS in our homes and things that are sometimes beyond our personal control.

Because we do not MOVE as much as our ancestors; we do not breathe as deeply as they did continuously while working harder physically.

We do not rest in natural rhythmical patterns because of artificial lighting.

We stress about everything if it does not immediately go exactly as we have planned it to go.

We use all the muscles in our bodies a lot less than our ancestors did.

In short, we are not living the same lifestyle our Scriptural ancestors did PHYSICALLY. And we are definitely are not living the same SPIRITUAL LIVES our spiritual ancestors lived.

THE PHYSICAL AND THE SPIRITUAL INTERTWINE

The Creator created mankind and set him in the perfect "terrarium". Every living thing could maintain and reproduce itself indefinitely before sin entered. After our first parent's sin, earth, animals, and man still could go on with all of their multitudes of perfect cycles except a few minor changes brought upon them by their sin. The elements then present could still feed, repair, and rebuild their injured bodies, however; just not eternally as first planned by our Father in Heaven.

Although the activities of man have increased, diversified, and become more complex, the BASIC NEEDS OF MAN ARE STILL THE SAME. Knowledge of the infinitely bigger and farther away and infinitely smaller has become better observed by man, but all the discoveries have only reinforced the things we knew all along- everything the Creator has created is wondrous, orderly, efficient, and constant.

If WE CAN ALWAYS RELY ON math principles in and of themselves and in all other sciences they permeate, electricity, the jet stream, ocean currents, magnetism, radio waves, chemistry, physics, hydrology, and other UNSEEN, BUT DEFINITELY POWERFUL FORCES put into effect at Creation, to affect our lives for the good when used with understanding, then we can also rely on the Creator's INVISABLE, ETERNAL, SPIRITUAL, and spiritual (CONDITIONAL)- that-affect-physical laws set up at Creation to be reliable and useful when used with understanding. Fighting these laws or rejecting them or neglecting them or polluting them physically will only bring us rebellion's reward—trouble, confusion, poor health, and possibly death. The Creator's invitation to "taste and see that the Creator is good" is an invitation to ALL He has to offer us. As we learn, change, obey, and incorporate ALL His commands into our lives, He blesses us more and more. We see the results of loving obedience to His loving instructions in the Torah.

The Creator's Word, the Scriptures, is like a banquet table the Creator lays out for all of us. Some people think they can pick and choose on that table, according to what pleases them. But the Creator's TRUE PEOPLE taste ALL He has for them, for on that table is all they MUST partake of to be called His child. Messiah said, "Man shall not live by bread alone, BUT BY EVERY WORD

THAT PROCEEDS OUT OF THE MOUTH OF THE CREATOR" (Matthew 4:4). Messiah also said only a few days before His passion, "The scribes and the Pharisees sit in Moses' seat: ALL THEREFORE WHATSOEVER THEY BID YOU OBSERVE, THAT OBSERVE AND DO" (Matthew 23:2, 3).

In other words, ALL of the Creator's commands and directions which apply directly to a PRESENT LIFE SITUATION are NECESSARY for us to INCORPORATE INTO OUR LIVES if we want the truly Creator blessed life. And ordering our health life after the Creator's plan is just ONE PART of this great plan for every aspect of our lives.

I will not spend a lot of time in this book telling you how man has spoiled our food, our water, our air, our environment, etc. for profit and personal pleasure. There are already many books that detail these things such as SILENT SPRING, DIET FOR A NEW AMERICA, MAD COWBOY, NO MORE BULL, ETC. We all already know that and mourn these facts.

I will not spend a great deal of time in this book telling you of the failures of the conventional INVENTED AND MANUFACTURED drug oriented medical health care system we have in modern society. We all have had very sick dear friends and relatives who became victims of the treatments that have brought further misery to these loved ones. The Hippocratic Oath, taken by every medical doctor, itself says, "First, do no harm." Nearly EVERY SINGLE CHEMICAL DRUG prescribed as "medicine" that is not found naturally occurring in food, herb, earth material, or body process, HAS SOME OR MANY HARMFUL SIDE EFFECTS!!!!! Does this in itself not send up red flags to anyone that something is not right here??

But what I do think the best conventional medicine has to offer right now is all the evaluating tests that are available to tell you WHAT you may have.

Emergency medicine has its benefits, also, because it can keep you alive, but it will NEVER improve your overall health. But it can keep you alive for ONE MORE CHANCE to help yourself get really healthy and stronger. This you can do by CHANGING HOW YOU TREAT YOUR BODY AND HOW YOU RELATE YOURSELF TO YOUR CREATOR!

It is also true, the reason that most western culture populations are living longer is probably because of the use of conventional antibiotics at the onset of normally devastating infections. In centuries past, if you got a bacterial infection, it was usually a death sentence for you. But each of these positive things comes with a price. Emergency room drugs can do great damage as well as save temporarily. Antibiotics disturb the functions of the protecting intestinal flora and can cause the occurrences of greater and more frequent infections in the future as well as hurting the actual functioning of the bowel and nervous system. At the same time, there are natural antibiotics that do no damage to the body and its functions.

THE HERBS AND HERBAL COMBINATIONS TOLD OF IN THIS BOOK HAVE THE CHEMICALS THE DRUG COMPANIES SAY THEY ARE LOOKING FOR TO CURE DIFFERENT DISEASES WITHOUT THE HARMFUL SIDE EFFECTS. I KNOW BECAUSE I HAVE USED THEM FOR YEARS WITH MY CLIENTS AND THEY WORK. THEY HEAL. THEY CURE. The drug companies should not seek that much to extract those chemicals to use as single compounds; they work better when taken with all the accompanying natural agents found in each herb. Instead, there should be a movement to grow MASSIVE square miles of organically grown medicinal herbs to be available for the sick and dying. There is a whole HUGE industry waiting to happen in this area for the bold and forward thinkers. To paraphrase some lines from the movie FORREST GUMP, "THERE ARE POWERED HERBS, CUT HERBS, HERB TEAS, HERB

TINCTURES, HERB COMBINATIONS, FRESH HERBS, ENCAPSULATED HERBS, CANCER HERBS, AIDS HERBS, DIABETES HERBS, ASTHMA HERBS, HERB SALVES, SEA HERBS, ETC. " You get the picture!

You should know that no drug company can get an exclusive patent on any naturally occurring chemical compound like ferrous sulfate (naturally occurring iron) or potassium iodide (a naturally occurring mucus dissolver) or sodium chloride (table salt, a natural cleanser). They can sell the naturally occurring chemicals (like bio-identical hormones), but have no exclusive corner of the drug market on them. They are always searching for chemicals THAT ARE NOT NATURALLY OCCURRING to get exclusive rights to to manufacture to boost their profits. This is why they formed deviations of natural substances like estrogen to sell. Their departure from nature has caused millions of women enormous harm.

As you view the healing choices you have, there is only so much you can do to change the vast number of things that are tearing your health down that are totally beyond your control. But there are CHANGES YOU CAN MAKE that ARE VERY MUCH UNDER YOUR CONTROL that will bring you back to good personal health if you are willing to be consistent, disciplined, and persistent to work on your problem.

The natural treatments I present here do not hurt the body, but in most cases, start SOOTHING, giving MORE ENERGY, and producing MORE of A FEELING OF WHOLENESS right from the start. Is this not what HEALING IS? To me, healing is a process that starts IMMEDIATELY when the right medicine or treatment is applied to the right condition that brings the individual back up to PERFECT health once again.

We have been DRUGGED (pun definitely intended!) into thinking, by huge drug companies, that all we should be looking for is a "better quality of life". We all tend to think within the parameters that as you age you should expect to get weaker and sicker and be on more and more drugs. This is not the SCRIPTURAL example at all. This is the manmade example.

When I am sick, I do not want just a better quality of life than I find myself in right now. I want ALL of my energy, ALL of my strength, ALL of my capabilities that I had before I was sick BECAUSE I KNOW IT IS POSSIBLE TO HAVE THAT!! I have experienced this many times, and I want to show you how you can have it, too.

The body has a wonderful capacity to perform perfectly when it is given every opportunity to do so. The Creator, in His infinite love and perfection, created it so. All the functions and chemical cycles of the body are programmed and ready to go if you only put the right elements in to run these processes. A sick body to me is like a car without the right gas and fluids. It is there all ready to perform. Although perfectly engineered, if it does not have the right gas and fluids to run the machine, it will not start and run properly. But, if the right gas and fluids are present, it runs PERFECTLY! If you have an old car with lots of gunk in the engine, you may have to take the time to clean out the gunk before it runs perfectly. But, as any good mechanic knows, if it is cleaned and tuned and filled with the right fluids, almost any car, no matter what the age, can run just like new time and time again. The body runs on like principles.

At the original writing of this book, I am 59 years old. I have been sick many times in my life. Strep throat, heart murmur, anemia, viral infections, fungal infections, a broken vertebrae, sun poisoning, mumps, measles, shingles, chigger bites, mosquito bite poisoning (over 50 bites at one time), Chagas disease, extreme tiredness from taking care of 8 children, the body stresses of

14 years straight of being either pregnant or nursing a baby (including twins!), dislocated vertebrae, scoliosis, 2 ripped rotator cuffs, infection in eye after tornado blown refuse landed in it, mold sinus infection, collapsed lung after severe blood loss of miscarriage, Asian flu, viruses, multiple parasite infections, toxoplasmosis, liver flukes, hookworms, round worms, pinworms, chemical toxic reactions, swollen lymph nodes, H1N1, mercury poisoning and chronic depression from amalgams, two near deadly poison ivy episodes including poison ivy in the lungs, undiagnosed hernia for 17 years, a nearly deadly MRSA infection, 3 months of viral pneumonia, black widow spider bite, and more I have experienced. Yet, today, I have more energy and feeling of well-being than I did as a normal teenager! Nearly each time I was able to overcome these problems with prayer and natural healing agents. From the time I gave my life over to the Creator at 18, I have used all natural remedies for most of the health problems I have faced. And the level of my health has only increased over the years using these wonderful things.

For anyone reading this book, I want to make it perfectly clear that in my understanding of health from a Scriptural perspective there is the possibility of divine, instantaneous healing performed in the name of the Messiah. I have prayed for others and they were instantaneously healed. It has occurred to me on 11 different occasions for 11 different conditions in my life at the writing of this book. At those times, there was no man, medicine, or money that could have helped me. I needed a true miracle. I called upon the Creator in the name of Messiah and He heard me and healed me. And I praise the Creator for that. But there have been other times when He showed me it is part of my daily faith-based obedience to take care of my body the same way we are to daily take care of the body of Messiah, the true believers. Just because He does not heal me instantaneously every time does not mean to me He has failed me or that my faith is too small for the task or that I have some hidden disobedience. I learned He has ALREADY graciously provided for my healing in the miraculous act of Creation things from the foundation of this Creation for me to use for my benefit.

My husband was an assistant pastor for several years. People would come to us or services we attended and ask for prayer for different health problems. Many times I thought, they do not need prayer; they need lifestyle changes. Sometimes I would gently suggest some changes that would help in the immediate and long-term future for their health problems. Most of the time, the suggestions and changes were ignored and sometime later, they would be back asking for prayer for the same problem or an EVEN GREATER problem! I often have wondered at these times, what does the loving, providing Creator think of this? To me, it is a form of laziness, deliberate ignorance, deliberate rebellion, or deliberate disobedience. They were just reaping rebellion's reward, especially after being given the answer on how to help their problem.

We will always be at the mercy of the physical elements of this world. A human WILL NEVER have the FULLNESS of the Creator driven part of the spiritual world interact in his physical life until 2 things are present – faith and obedience. Deuteronomy 27-30 shows us this very plainly. This law of living in this life is so distinctly stated in these 4 chapters. Our Father in Heaven gives us very specific indicators of our level of faith and obedience and their rewards or punishments that it leaves no gray areas. Read this with the most transparent heart and see where you fall. If you have faith (and I believe most people in most churches do) and you are not receiving ALL His benefits and protections, it is time to check your obedience level. By the way, this is something the devil does not want you to do BECAUSE THAT WAS HIS FAILURE and not doing it is his deception!!!

We have been told erroneously that the Creator's laws are not applicable today. Have the laws of hydrology been done away ? Have the laws of physics or chemistry been done away? Did pigs change their nature at the cross? Did mathematics laws change at the cross? Messiah said none of the laws of the Creator in Matthew 5:17-19 would be obliterated until heaven and earth pass. ALL these laws were set up at Creation. The laws of the Creator show us how to live in the most blessed state or highest level in this life. Although they were on different levels, they are all the Creator's laws and will be with us and affect us and govern us until heaven and earth pass. The only times we will see a shift in these is when a MIRACLE is done on the wonderful rare occasions when the Creator decides to let His overwhelming POWER AND LOVE be shown. I have seen it many times myself, but I also know we dare not be presumptuous on the daily housekeeping of our body.

It is not just wisdom you need. It is not just knowledge you need. It is not just prayer you need. It is not just faith you need. It is not just laying on of hands you need. It is not just anointing you need. You need action and obedience, too. Faith without works is DEAD.

Many die from lack of knowledge. Many also die from lack of motivation or laziness.

The first publicly recorded words of both John the Baptist and messiah were "REPENT". Repent means change. Change means on every level that affects you and separates you from the Creator and all His will for you to live the best life! You will receive freedom when you repent of all the ways that are tearing you from the Creator and His ways. The truth will set you free when you seek, find, knock, learn, acknowledge, and incorporate truth into every area of your life.

Faith and faith-based obedience go hand in hand. It is action as opposed to in-action into the Creator's approved ways. You can not get the fullness of life in every area of your life He promises until you surrender and actually CHANGE your way of doing things into doing them the Creator's way. He says He gives His spirit to them who OBEY Him (Acts 5:32). Why would He give His Spirit to them who disobey Him? There is a spirit there, for sure, but it is not the Spirit of the Creator. Would that TRULY bring honor to His name and cause?

Deuteronomy 27-30 is an exceptionally revealing part of the Scriptures in another way, also. It reveals also the point at which the physical world or realm intersects the spiritual realm. It shows a mere human how to get the CONTINUAL (WITHOUT INTERRUPTION) intervention of the Heavenly Father in his life. It reveals the physical as well as the spiritual well-beings and their wellsprings. It all comes from faith and obedience on your part for the Heavenly Father to turn on the faucet JUST FOR YOU AND ALL YOUR VERY SPECIFIC NEEDS.

CHAPTER 2

HOW DO WE GET SICK?

Unless you were born with a missing part or with a genuine genetic defect that shows up from the day of birth, you were born an individually encapsulated energy-producing organism called a human. Mother's milk and a mother's love, protection from the elements, and frequent bathing was all you needed to survive. You had perfect health and grew healthily and quickly. Then, one day, this perfectly healthy human got sick. Something was wrong. Something interrupted this human's perfect health. What was it?

In my study of health from a Scriptural, scientific point of view, I have found there are only certain things that can make a perfectly healthy physical body sick or not function to its fullest capacity. These are...

PARASITES AND OTHER LIVING MICROORGANISMS

VIRUSES

BACTERIA

MOLDS

FUNGI

CHEMICAL POLLUTANTS

MALNUTRITION BECAUSE OF STRESS (GOOD OR BAD DIET, BAD MANAGEMENT)

MALNUTRITION CAUSED FROM FAULTY DIET (JUST BAD DIET)

OVER-NUTRITION (TOO MUCH FOOD)

DELIBERATE DISOBEDIENCE OF ANY OF THE CREATOR'S WORD

DEMONIC MIMICING OF ANY POOR HEALTH CONDITION KNOWN TO MAN

LACK OF SUNLIGHT

LACK OF WATER (DEHYDRATION OR UNCLEANLINESS)

LACK OF REST

LACK OF MODERATION

LACK OF FRESH AIR

LACK OF MINIMAL EXERCISE

LACK OF SANITATION

Or a combination of any of the above!

Now this may seem very elementary to everyone, but modern drug driven medicine does not always believe this or run its researches on these facts. It makes up chemical combinations to COMBAT, LOGJAM, INTERRUPT, OR STOP THE SYMPTOMS of the presence of one or several of the above without acknowledging that any of the above (or combinations of the above) is directly CAUSING the condition or work toward the elimination of the cause.

They have the right idea in one case – they think the cure is in a chemical reaction. This is partly true. Most disruptions in the smooth running of the body are a disruption of a chemical process. The real answer, however, is in finding what is CAUSING the chemical reaction to be disrupted, not adding another foreign chemical for the body to deal with.

To understand how to combat or correct these things, we first must understand what concern the Creator has for our health. We need to understand what HE says we need to do to get good health.

CHAPTER 3

THE CREATOR'S CONCERN FOR OUR HEALTH

It is the Creator's will we be in good health. He wants us to have CONTINUAL, GOOD HEALTH.

1.

"Beloved, I wish above all things that thou mayest prosper and be in health, even as thy soul prospereth." 3 John 2

"That Thy way may be known upon the earth, Thy saving health among ALL nations." Psalms 67:2

2.

It is our responsibility to take good care of our bodies for the Messiah's sake. Many people use their bodies like A DIXIE CUP... JUST USE IT AND THROW IT AWAY. But we should use it like A LIBRARY BOOK...USE IT AND RETURN IT IN AS GOOD OF CONDITION AS POSSIBLE!

"Know ye not that ye are the temple of the Creator, and that the Spirit of the Creator dwelleth in you? If any man defile the temple of the Creator, him shall the Creator destroy: for the temple of the Creator is HOLY, which temple ye are." 1 Corinthians 3:16, 17

"For no man ever yet hated his own flesh: but nourisheth and cherisheth it, even as the Messiah the church." Ephesians 5:9

"For ye are bought with a price: therefore glorify the Creator in your body, and in your spirit, which are the Creator's." 1 Corinthians 6:20

"Whether therefore ye eat, or drink, or whatsoever ye do, do all to the glory of the Creator." 1 Corinthians 10:31

3.

The Creator has commanded us from creation what we may and may not eat, starting with instruction to Adam and Eve in the Garden of Eden. He made a separation between what was permissible and good for us and what was not permissible and harmful for us.

"And the Creator commanded the man, saying, Of every tree of the garden thou mayest freely eat: But of the tree of the knowledge of good and evil, thou shalt not eat of it: for in the day that thou eatest thereof thou shalt surely die." Genesis 2:16, 17

"And the Creator said, Behold, I have given you every green herb bearing seed, which is upon the face of all earth, and every green tree, in the which is the fruit of a tree yielding seed: to you it shall be meat (food)." Genesis 1:29

"Thou shalt eat the herb of the field." Genesis 3:18

4.

The knowledge of which animals were acceptable and were not acceptable as food and sacrifices was known before Moses' time by Noah. Although some think no meat was eaten before the flood, still the distinction of which animals were acceptable as sacrifices and labeled as clean or unclean was known by

Noah and most likely from Creation by Adam. There were seven times as many clean animals taken into the Ark as unclean animals.

"Of every clean beast thou shalt take to thee by sevens, the male and his female; and of the beasts that are not clean by two, the male and his female.'
Genesis 7:2

5.

The Creator allowed Moses to write down specific names of animals that we are permitted to eat as food. All other animals are considered off limits as food and designed by the Creator for another purpose in creation. These unclean animals or scavengers or predators are the garbage collectors of the earth. They help keep the earth and our environment clean by consuming and encapsulating the dead and decaying filth of the earth from plant and animal sources in their bodies for our protection. It is DEADLY to consume these animals as their filth passes to our body upon eating them. The strongest word of disgust (abomination) found in Scripture is used in reference to using these unclean animals for food.

Leviticus 11 and Deuteronomy 14:1-21
Read whole chapters for complete details

Beasts we may eat must be cloven footed (splits the hoof) and must chew the cud-examples-cow, sheep, goat, deer, moose, elk, buffalo, bison, etc.
Beasts we MAY NOT EAT –
Examples- hog, pig, raccoon, squirrel, rabbit, bear, etc.

Swimming water animals (fish) we may eat must have fins and scales

Examples- cod, flounder, salmon, tuna, mahi mahi, whitefish, haddock. etc.

We MAY NOT EAT-

Examples- squid, shrimp, scallops, clams, lobster, crab, shark, etc.

Birds we may eat

Examples- chicken, turkey, pigeon, dove, etc.

Birds we MAY NOT EAT-

Examples- owl, raven, eagle, swan, bat, etc.

Bugs we may eat

Examples- locusts, beetles, grasshoppers, etc.

Animals WE MAY NOT EAT

Examples- weasels, anything with paws, anything that flies having four feet, mice, lizards, snail, mole, etc.

Even in the NEW TESTAMENT we are told not to touch unclean things. "Wherefore come out from among them, and be ye separate, saith the Creator, and touch not the UNCLEAN THING; and I will receive you". 2 Corinthians 6:17

Unclean birds are still considered unclean in the book of Revelation telling of happenings to come to pass at the end of this age-"...a cage of every unclean and hateful bird." Revelation 18:2

Isaiah prophesies that the Creator will destroy THOSE LIVING AT THE TIME OF MESSIAH'S SECOND COMING who are eating swine's flesh, mice, and the abomination (ANY UNCLEAN ANIMAL)- Leviticus 11 and Deuteronomy 14:3; Isaiah 66:17

6.

The Creator forbids us the following things for our good and health-

Blood and animal fats

Leviticus 3:17; 7:23, 24; 17:10, 14

Animal fat clogs the arteries and blood carries many diseases. Blood also carries the very life of the flesh.

We are to be married to and limit our sexual experiences to only one person at a time for life, and, it is preferred that both partners be virgins. This eliminates the possibilities of sexually transmitted diseases being transmitted in the population. Matthew 19:5

7.

The Creator instructs us on many levels on issues that affect our health.

We are to be moderate and temperate in our lifestyles.

Philippians 4:5

We are not to overeat, be drunk, or worry.

Luke 21:34

We are to limit even our honey consumption.

Proverbs 25:16

We are to use the herbs for our health and help.

Psalms 104:14

Fermented grape juice may be used as a stomach remedy.

1 Timothy 5:23

Figs may be used as a boil remedy.

Isaiah 38:21

Wine and oil may be used to heal open and closed wounds.

Luke 10:34

In the future, leaves of the tree of life will heal the nations.

Revelation 22:2

All male babies are to be circumcised on the 8th day of life

8.

There are several avenues of the Heavenly Father's approved healing.

OBEDIENCE AND MERCY

Obeying ALL of the Creator's commands (The Torah), being merciful, recognizing truth, trusting in the Creator, fearing the Creator, and departing from evil will bring about good health.

Proverbs 3:1-8

Being merciful to other people and keeping the Creator's commandments, including His holy Sabbath days, will bring about healing.

Isaiah 58:1-14

ONE OF THE MOST IMPORTANT STATEMENTS IN THIS BOOK!

People do not realize that excellent health ESCAPES THEM FOR THESE ABOVE REASONS ALONE AT TIMES!!!!

NATURAL METHODS-REST

Daily rest, adequate sleep in total darkness (no nightlights!) - even the Messiah had to rest. Dr. Peter Maas and other sleep researchers have found the brain and body can not fully heal, recuperate, and permanently imprint new knowledge unless we sleep in total darkness for about 7 hours!

Mark 6:31

Researchers have discovered that most of your body's healing goes on when you are asleep!

Losing sleep makes your immune system go into overdrive by multiplying white blood cells up to 11 times over normal count!

Weekly rest, the seventh day Sabbath

Exodus 20:8-11

Hebrews 4:4-10

Isaiah 58: 13, 14

Two week long vacations a year where any Creator approved food desired may be consumed. The spring feast commands that no leaven (yeast based) be consumed for the week long feast. This helps clear the system of possible related yeast infections!

Leviticus 23

NATURAL METHODS-EXERCISE

Exercise keeps circulation open, posture straight, lymph system draining, cerebral fluids from pooling, organs functioning, bowel elimination regular, muscles strong to keep bones straight, dispels depression by the production of mood elevating chemicals, and many other health benefits. Exercise is one answer to depression, along with regualrly eating enough.

1 Kings 19:1-18

NATURAL METHODS-PROPER EATING

The eating of all natural organic foods, the use of herbs, vitamins, minerals, specific foods for specific conditions, eliminating harmful substances in foods, and eliminating forbidden substances will all help in bringing about more strength and a higher level of health. Ecclesiastes 10:17

NATURAL METHODS-FASTING AND MODERATION

Both fasting and exercising moderation in all things you do allow the body to rest, not be overtaxed, and allow time for recuperation and elimination.

Philippians 4:5

NATURAL METHODS-FRESH AIR AND SUNSHINE

Fresh air brings additional oxygen to the body. It also contains ozone, and positive and negative ions that all help disinfect the lungs and body. Sunshine produces vitamin D, which strengthens bones, and serotonin, which dispels depression. Direct sunlight also kills some pathogens on contact. Sunshine also raises the body temperature slightly, further killing some pathogens inside the body. Everyone should spend AT LEAST one half hour in the fresh air and sunshine every day. Fresh air should be available all night while sleeping, also.

NATURAL METHODS-WATER

The body, being made up of over 75% water, needs a fresh supply regularly internally. It is also very important to use fresh water on the OUTSIDE of the body to constantly wash off the multitudes of pathogens that land on it every day. Exodus 29:4

NATURAL METHODS- CLEANLINESS OF LIVING AREA

The home you continually dwell in must be kept very clean with the natural disinfectants and cleansers of water, apple cider vinegar, lemon juice, baking soda, borax, orange oil, and grapefruit seed extract, pine oil, solution of myrrh, and ammonia, etrog (Israel's wild lemon), etc. Leviticus 13:54

NATURAL METHODS-STRESS MANAGEMENT

Trusting in the Creator for everything, using your time wisely, getting enough rest, exercising, trusting those who have proven themselves reliable in the past to help you, forgiving those who are not as perfect as you are ☺, remembering that the Creator promises to help us when we endeavor to do our best—all of these things help to beat stress. Titus 3:2; Proverbs 3:5

NATURAL METHODS-PROPER DRESS

It is very important to your health to dress properly. In the cold weather, the body should be dressed warmly enough to keep a warm and even body temperature. In the warm weather, the clothes should be loose, light, but modest, to keep the direct sunlight off the body for most of the day. The arm from elbow to shoulder and the leg from knee to hip are part of the regulating thermostat of the body. These body parts should be modestly clothed at ALL times, appropriate to weather conditions to maintain even body temperatures. This is just another benefit to obeying the Creator's command to be modestly dressed that few people are aware of. 1Timothy 2:9

Use single fiber clothing. Each fiber has its own temperature controlling factors such as wicking, weight, density, etc. Deuteronomy 22:11

Women should wear single natural fiber clothing that is loose (skirts or dresses) around the pelvic area for air flow to prevent urinary and reproductive congestion and infections. Deuteronomy 22:5

Shoes should be of natural materials and as flat to the ground as possible to mimic walking barefoot. Balance, posture affecting internal organs' functioning and back support, heavy metal exposure by touching synthetic leathers, and proper sufficient width are all factors to be considered when purchasing shoes.

SPIRITUAL METHODS-PRAYER AND FASTING TO REMOVE DEMONIC INFLUENCES

The devil and his demons can bring upon a human any disease or condition produced by pathogens. He is a copycat. Exodus 7:10, 11; 7: 20-22; 8:6, 7 The Messiah said some conditions that affect the body will ONLY go out by prayer and fasting. Matthew 17:21; Mark 9:29

SPIRITUAL METHODS- PRAYER, LYING ON OF THE HANDS AND ANOINTING BY THE ELDERS, VOCAL REBUKING, AND TALLIT USE

Our forefathers had a great knowledge of the use of essential oils for healing along with prayer.

"Is any sick among you? Let him call for the elders of the church; and let them pray over him, anointing him with oil in the name of the Messiah: And the prayer of faith shall save the sick, and the Messiah shall raise him up; and if he has committed sins, they shall be forgiven him." James 5:14

Laying on of the hands for miraculous, instantaneous healing - Matthew 9:18; Mark 5:23; Mark 16:18; Mark 6:5; Luke 4:40; Luke 13:13; Acts 28:8

Rebuking by vocal, faith filled command aimed at the disease, the devil that caused the disease, or the injured body part – Matthew 17:18; Mark 1:25; Mark 9:25; Luke 4:35; Luke 4:39; Luke 9:42

Wrapping the sick in tallits (prayer shawls with blue fringes or tassels OR TZITZIT) and praying with touching the sick body parts with the tassels. Matthew 14:36; Malachi 4:2

This refers to the healing in his "wings" (tassels or fringes) predicted by Malachi of Messiah and the healings that happened as people touched His tzitzits.

CHAPTER 4

HOW DO WE GET WELL?

THERE IS A FULL FLEDGED WAR GOING ON CONTINUALLY INSIDE AND
OUTSIDE OF YOUR BODY ON YOUR HEALTH. You must declare full out and
out war in return on it. One change usually will not bring about the high level
of health you are looking for. MANY CHANGES in lifestyle will be needed to get
the level of health you desire because true health is a package deal. Your will
and your body are in a war for survival on a daily basis. If you want full,
bursting health, you are going to have to declare full, all out war on every
aspect that is tearing it down. The more changes you make and the more
quickly you make them, the faster your health will return and increase to the
high level of health you desire. This is a type of REPENTANCE...changing over
to doing things the right way!

Your grandmother and mother may have taught you one way of eating or living,
but you are personally responsible to do things the Creator's way whether they
did it that way or not! Erroneous habits can be broken with the Creator's great
power available at your disposal.

Your parents or grandparents may have or MAY live longer than you ever will
BECAUSE of all the factors that are present now that can tear your health
down that THEY NEVER HAD TO FACE! Only if you make a directed effort to
do the best you can to change as many things as you can will you have a
greater chance at better health.

The body is such a marvelous creation. Just as the Creator through the angels,
and the Holy Spirit are working every day to help you survive this life
spiritually, guiding and protecting you, the Creator has designed the body to

fight constantly for your physical life on many fronts, even if you do not acknowledge Him. There is mercy and love abounding in this keeping you alive and functioning, giving you more time on earth to find Him, acknowledge Him, live for Him, and receive every good blessing He has in store for you in faith and obedience. Every day, every hour, and every minute of your life it is fighting for survival. It is fighting multitudes of microbes 24 hours a day while trying to perform its normal duties of nourishing you, keeping all your organs and other functions running smoothly, keeping your brain bright and cheerful thinking, keeping your body temperature steady, keeping your heart beating, and eliminating anything that is not useful to the body. Those days you feel a little bit more tired than usual, it is in overdrive, fighting a battle for your survival. You need to use every thing at your disposal to improve your health and increase your chances of achieving the best health!

EAT REAL ORGANIC FOOD

One of the most important paragraphs in this book is the following----

Every time you put any non-food in your body (such as junk foods, half foods, fractionated foods, alternative foods, fake foods, or chemically laden foods) and hope to get some energy from those foods, it has to work even HARDER because you have not given it the materials to fight off the very thing you have put into it! This alone will give you a whole new perspective on what really IS food. You cannot get energy or healing from a substance that the body has to work hard to eliminate. Anything put in the body the body is not Creator programmed to use as food has to use lots of energy and stored good chemicals (beneficial nutrients) to analyze and eliminate. That is why eating non-foods and half foods (soda, white flour, white rice, sugar, Sugar, SUGAR, artificial colors, artificial flavors, conventional herbicides and pesticides, etc.) tear down your health and leave you feeling depressed and weak. They add nothing to your storehouse of good chemicals to use in emergencies, and they draw from what reserves you may have to help eliminate it. Soon you have nothing to fight with, nothing to build with, nothing to repair with, and no energy production.

It dumbfounds me that I should have to mention in a book on regaining health that the very basis for recovering good health is eating REAL WHOLE ORGANIC FOOD. When did we ever stop eating REAL FOOD? It was at this point that all these CONFOUNDING modern diseases started becoming apparent and widespread.

I truly believe that the devil himself is behind all the non-foods we are eating. It is a deception that people think anything offered as food is really food. ONLY REAL ORGANIC FOOD is real food for the body. The food given to mankind in the Garden of Eden was organic, fresh, ripe, local, and, in most cases, raw!

EAT ONLY ORGANIC FOODS, JUICES, AND HERB TEAS

The very basis of good health is eating REAL WHOLE ORGANIC FOODS. It is the basement, the cellar, the felt board, the chalkboard, and the very foundation upon which good health rests. Plainly grown foods in an organic, untouched, and uncontaminated manner is still, and always was, the best way to grow and eat foods. It was the Creator's simple plan from the beginning that mankind tend gardens with the natural materials at hand in the yearly pattern. It will SOON BE the main occupation of the millennium! (Isaiah 2:4; Joel 3:10; Micah 4:3)

The only way to completely nourish the body is to eat organically grown foods in their whole state. Eating an apple is better for you than drinking apple juice.

Eating whole wheat flour is better than eating just the white part white flour. Eating a whole potato is better than French fries or just the white part of the potato. There is a spiritual lesson in this, too. Tasting and seeing the Creator is good in all aspects of your life...taking in all of what He ask us to do and experience...gives us a fuller life-the life in abundance Messiah spoke of.

AND-the best way to consume foods is raw. To recover your health, you must eat many of your foods raw. These live foods have enzymes that help the body clean and restore body functions back to normal. There is no substitute for raw organic foods in restoring health!

A simple, whole foods organic diet, even if monotonous, is better for you than a varied diet including junk food. The spiritual lesson here is that doing what is right in some areas mixed in with doing what is wrong and sinning in other areas still adds up to an unrighteous life. If you break one rule of health, you will reap the reward of breaking them all, also. But doing ALL of what is right and pleasing and commanded by the Creator brings ever-flowing peace and blessing. And uninterrupted good health!!

There are many places you can buy real food. Most supermarkets now have sections of naturally grown or organic foods. There are several nationwide (in the USA) chains like Whole Foods, Earth Fare, etc. and locally owned individual health food stores that have everything you need to get started. These can be used as your main grocery store. There are many mail order houses that sell raw, natural, and organic foods on the Internet, also, such as Vitacost.com, and nuts.com. There are also local ORGANIC farmers everywhere who are willing to sell their extra produce to you. Most states have a listing of all the organic farmers in their state listed on the Internet. There are local food co-ops that you and some friends can organize that buy organic foods in bulk and split the food up among the members at meetings. There are also farmers' markets popping up in nearly every small town now. And you can always grow it yourself! Buying from a local organic farmer's market or growing food yourself are your best and cleanest sources for your food supply.

Right now one of the greatest services a church member can do for the people in their congregation and community is to grow organic food for the members to buy. It is one very important link in the continuing service for the Creator. Considering that organic food was the ONLY kind of food you could buy up until about 75 years ago, and considering what a rarity it can be in some areas to find a steady supply of organic foods, it is a very valuable service rendered. Opening a small health food store or organic produce stand where all of these foods can be obtained and where local farmers can sell their produce is another great service to the local congregation and the community. Opening a small organic, vegetarian restaurant is another invaluable service to the community. I know of a church that maintains a huge organic garden IN ITS VAST CHURCH LAWN for all of its members and the poor. Many people SHARE THE WORK in this garden AND MANY MORE BENEFIT FROM IT!

Your first choice for food should be---ORGANIC, FRESH, RAW, and RIPE

Your second choice for food should be—ORGANIC, RAW, RIPE, and DRIED

Your third choice for food should be—ORGANIC, RAW, RIPE, and FROZEN

Your fourth choice for food should be--- ORGANIC, COOKED

Raw foods contain live enzymes that CONSTANTLY HEAL AND CLEANSE THE BODY. Cooked food has lost all enzyme activity, but still has some nutritional value. Foods that are frozen are very health building if frozen when raw. Freezing, however, destroys most Vitamin B-6 and Vitamin E in the food, 2 things needed for the health and life of the heart. Beans must be cooked to be digestible. Their main value is minerals and protein. NEVER EAT SPROUTS but do eats shoots or microgreens!! More on that later in the book!

Many complain that buying organic foods is too expensive. My reply is yes and no. If you stop buying all the junk food and sink that amount of money into whole, organic foods, you will see you will have money left over.

I feel you pay for non-foods, junk foods, fake foods, alternative foods, chemically laden foods, and half foods 3 TIMES- FIRSTLY at the check-out, SECONDLY at the doctor for random, year in and year out infections and health problems, and THIRDLY AND LASTLY on your death bed, when you SPEND MOST OF THE MONEY YOU COULD HAVE LEFT FOR AN INHERITANCE on trying to save your life from a life of poor eating and poor care of your body. So you see, in the end, buying organic foods is MUCH cheaper! And you just feel better many more days of your life using organic foods.

I think, from all my experience with people who have been desperately sick, you can not afford NOT to eat all organic all of the time!

Organic foods are the basis of a health building and health sustaining real foods lifestyle diet, but there are more things you should know in the next chapter.

CHAPTER 5

THINGS YOU NEED TO KNOW BEFORE YOU START REBUILDING YOUR
HEALTH!

You have or maybe a friend of yours has just gotten the bad news from the
doctor. You have a disease for which at this point conventional medicine has
no cure. You are shocked. You are angry. You are confused. You are very
panicky. You feel very alone and powerless. You feel depressed beyond your
deepest depression ever.

You had a friend, or your parents HAD a friend, who had the very same disease
you are now said to have. They died what you would class as a terrible death.
The doctors gave them treatments that robbed them of life, vigor, and dignity.
The treatments seemed just as bad, if not worse, than the silent disease they
had. Secretly, you feel everyone who knew this person felt the person would
have been better off if they had not had the treatments and had just died a
natural, progressing death. You wonder how, with all the money being pumped
into research for this disease for so many long years, doctors have not
discovered what really causes it and what really permanently cures it.

You remember hearing the doctors told this person there was a 20% chance of
this or a 45% chance of that if they took the conventional cure. Right now, you
don't want to hear percentages. You want to know how to completely rid
yourself of this corpse-like condition that you are now dragging around with
you day and night as soon as possible. You are absolutely loath to spend every
single dollar you have accumulated up to this point on a percentage that may
not be on your side that could possibly go to your children, or that could help
someone in the future as an endowment or missionary effort.

On top of all of that, you are thinking…. I should have had more children; I should have been nicer to my mother. I should have gotten a spiritual life somewhere along the line, because, boy, it looks like I am going to need it.

A Parable

You need a new car. You know exactly the type you need and want that will fill all your needs. All you want is a good model to just be able to go to work each day and provide for your family for a long time. Everyone, as far as you know, in town goes to the same dealership in town to get a new car. You walk in with $20,000. cash in your hand that you have worked very hard and long to save to buy a car that you can enjoy for years of good service.   When you start to sign the agreement to buy the beautiful car you have picked out and hand over your money, the salesman tells you that you have a 20% to 45% chance of receiving 20% to 45% of the car you just ordered. Not only that, you will also have to leave some of your clothing on the dealership floor before they let you go out the door. You know there is NO WAY you can go very far in life without all of your clothes. You are absolutely stunned and embarrassed that you could be so taken in and that no one has had the guts to expose the foolhardiness of their business dealings.

But, a close friend that you have always felt was really straight and truthful with you in the past, tells you of another dealership in the area that not many people know about. They sell the very car you want for about $1,000. They promise delivery within 3 months or so. This friend knows several people who have purchased from this dealership, and this dealership has delivered on its promises, and they are now the proud owners of the FULL car of their dreams. And they did not have to leave their clothes anywhere! You decide to think about purchasing a car from this dealership. You tell several of your friends that you have heard of another dealership where you can get just what you almost spent $20,000. on for only $1,000. And you can get ALL of it, FOR SURE, in about 3 months. One friend says you are crazy. Another friend says everybody in town always uses the first dealership—why do you have to be different? Another friend tells you not to trust the second dealership, even though this friend has never heard of it or investigated it or known anyone who has purchased from this dealership. One of your relatives begs you not to go to the second dealership as she is sure you will lose your $1,000. and never get your car and you will eventually have to go to the first dealership anyway.

In spite of all these things, you really know that there is no way you will ever gamble your $20,000. with even a chance of losing it or its buying power in a more used situation. And you certainly are not going to leave any of your clothes anywhere! And you are not going to be fooled or shanghaied. You ask your close friend to please introduce you to some of the people he knows who have purchased from the second dealership. You meet them and see their beautiful cars. They tell you it is really true they only spent $1,000. on their cars. They show you their bank accounts where they each still have $19,000. left. You decide to purchase from the second dealership in spite of all your friends' fears, suspicions, ignorance, and discouragements. And you get your car in about 3 months, all of it, and it lasts you for a very long time. Longer than all the cars of all the people that did not want you to purchase it at the second dealership. And you still have $19,000. in the bank.

Do you get it? Hear the parable of the car dealership! The car is your health. The money is what you spent on it. The percentages are what you REALLY get! The first dealership is conventional medicine. The second dealership is all natural medicine. The clothes are parts of your body. The friend is reason, truth, and facts. The $19,000. is, well, $19,000!

You are about to start a plan to regain your health. You have decided to take your health future in your own hands. One pill or one herb will not reverse a problem that has most likely taken years to develop. Remember! In order to regain your full health and strength, you must decide to declare full, all-out war on this condition. The more changes you make for the better toward reversing this condition, the faster and more likely you will actually be able to overcome this condition. Good health is a total lifestyle. Start today! You can do this! Thousands of others already have and have come out to be...HEALTHY AND WHOLE!

In order to drastically improve your health, there are going to be some things you must ADD YOUR LIFE and some things you must ELIMINATE FROM YOUR LIFE. This holds true also when you enter a spiritual life. There are areas where you will have to add some things you have never known or practiced before to start living a godly life. There will also be some things from your former life you are going to have to eliminate from your life to live pleasing to your Creator. Both actions in both cases bring you back to NORMAL, HEALTHY, WHOLENESS, AND YOUR CREATOR'S ORIGINAL PLAN FOR YOUR GOOD in your health life and spiritual life!

The following few chapters are a quick review of several essential things that must be addressed before full health can be restored from a nutritional and digestive point of view.

CHAPTER 6

EAT ONLY ORGANICALLY GROWN FOODS, THE ORIGINAL AND ONLY REAL FOOD

The only food EVER intended as fuel for the human body is organically grown food. The foods in the Garden of Eden were organically grown. Most foods available to humans up until around 1940 were ONLY organically grown. This, to most people, seems very simple and logical, but look at what most people, especially in the USA, are regularly devouring. There are said to be over 10,000 non-food origin chemicals (chemicals not naturally occurring in a naturally grown food, earth material, mineral or plant origin) available to be put on our foods from before the seeds are planted in the ground until you eat it off your plate. These non-food origin chemicals slow down, stop, or logjam many of the normally progressive chemical processes in our body. When this happens, the body cannot work or repair as it should. By eating only whole, organically grown foods, you eliminate these foreign chemicals as well as provide for the body the complete fuel and abundant nourishment it needs to continue functioning in a normal manner.

Of these 10,000 possible chemicals that can be applied to our foods, there are 400 that are the most commonly used and consumed in our foods. There has not been even ONE study to evaluate the interaction of even 2 of these chemicals, let alone the possible interactions of 400 times 400 interactions and reactions that could possibly be occurring in your body. No wonder there are times we just do not feel right or well!

Of course, when we talk about this "organic food' category it also includes herbs and essential oils used as medicine.

Every time you eat a food with pesticides, herbicides, or any chemical on it that was never intended by the Creator to enter your digestive system, you are slowly poisoning yourself and weakening your body for tomorrow. You reap what you sow.

Would you pick an apple off a tree, spray it with pest spray, and then eat it? Most likely not if you had to apply it yourself. Yet, when you eat conventionally grown produce, you could be eating 2 to 10 layers of different sprays on the individual fruit or vegetable. If you eat several fruits or vegetables at one meal, you could be taking in 2 to 30 types of pesticides or herbicides PER MEAL!

Most non-food chemicals applied to foods are accumulated in your tissues, and especially your liver. This cumulative effect, as time passes, allows your body to get weaker and weaker and more susceptible to various health problems.

Pesticides usually work on the nervous or digestive system of the insect. Maybe that is why we have more nerve problems, muscle pain, and digestive problems than EVER in our society.

A study at the University of Pennsylvania recently showed that organically grown foods have 100 to 1,000 times the BENEFICIAL nutrient content of conventionally grown foods at the same calorie content. And they do not have harmful chemicals attached to them that your body must fight with to eliminate from your system.

You need organically grown foods, which have higher nutrient content, more than conventionally grown foods to eliminate the HARMFUL chemicals you have eaten in the past that have been in the conventionally grown foods!!

You can not get energy, growth, or repair from a "food' that is contaminated or has applied chemicals in it that need to be eliminated from the body upon digestion.

From 47 years of experience, I have seen that the body cannot FULLY AND PERMANENTLY RECOVER FROM ANY HEALTH PROBLEM unless organic foods are the foundation of the diet. BECAUSE OF THE VAST AND VARIED DAMAGE ALL THESE CHEMICALS CAN DO (WE ARE SLOWLY DISCOVERING), EVERY MOTHER IN AMERICA SHOULD BE CHANTING "ORGANIC NOW! ORGANIC NOW!" TO AMERICA'S GROWERS FOR HER UNPROTECTED CHILD'S PRESENT AND FUTURES' SAKE! ORGANIC NOW!

AND MOST OF THAT ORGANIC WHOLE FOOD SHOULD BE IN ITS RAW AND RIPE STATE!

NOTE! GMO FOODS ARE NOT NATURAL TO THE BODY .THEY ARE GENETICALLY MODIFIED TO INCLUDE DNA AND OTHER CHEMICAL PARTS OF OTHER ORGANISMS.THEY PRODUCE TUMORS IN LAB ANIMALS.THEY ARE DIFFERENT FROM NATURALLY OCCURRING HYBRIDS WHICH YOUR BODY CAN USE EASILY.JUST ANOTHER REASON TO GO ORGANIC!

CHAPTER 7

ELIMINATE ALLERGIC OR INTOLERATED FOODS TEMPORARILY

You may notice that some foods, though whole and organic, just do not seem to give you energy. If you are eating small quantities and eating a great variety of foods and still know that some foods seem to take away your energy instead of giving you energy, leave that food alone for awhile. Until your body gets stronger and until maybe your blood is cleaner, you may have an intolerance or slight allergy to that food. That allergy or intolerance may have come from consuming that food too regularly by not switching the variety of foods you eat. As you build your whole system back up to normal health and strength, you will soon be able to tolerate almost any whole organic vegan food very well IN MODERATION.

The only exceptions to the above paragraph are the use of dairy and gluten products. A great proportion of the population is intolerant to cow dairy products and gluten containing grains. To find out if you are one of these people, leave them totally alone for one month and evaluate how you feel. Almost everyone I have suggested try this trial has decided to FOREVER STOP OR SEVERELY LIMIT their consumption of cow dairy and gluten products because of the improvement of their energy and health problems.

Another consideration is the use of GMO foods. If you eat organic foods, they most likely will not be GMO foods in the USA. These GMO foods are genetically modified and not natural as foods for the body. Eliminate these from your diet and many of your symptoms will resolve quickly!

CHAPTER 8

DRINK AND WASH IN PURE WATER

Water molecules, as we all know, are made of two hydrogen atoms and one oxygen atom. The form of water that truly hydrates and cleanses the body is in the penta-hydrate form. This form is a ring of 5 water molecules. It is estimated that pre-flood (in Noah's time) water had about 50% to 85% penta-hydrate form water in it. Today's tap water has about 2% penta-hydrate form brought about by the breakdown of this form by acid rain and other pollutants. Recent findings revealed recycled city water had many drug residues in it. 100% organic fruit and vegetable juices, especially freshly made organic juices, contain about 50% to 85% penta-hydrate form water. In critical and chronic cases, I urge my clients to drink plenty of freshly made ORGANIC fruit and vegetable juices, Prima plant based bottled water, commercially prepared penta-hydrate water, OR, at the very least, distilled water only, 6 or 8 stage filtered water, or ZERO filter water.

There are literally thousands of pathogens landing on your skin and hair from the air, from people breathing, coughing, sneezing near you, from what you touch everyday, from the wind blowing, and even from the flushing action of your toilet! Showering every day at least once removes these accumulated pathogens and the oils that can make them "stick" to your skin. Use a very simple organic formula PH balanced soap that is gentle on the skin.

Showering is preferable over a tub bath as the shower flushes the pathogens away from the hair and skin while a tub bath allows you to soak in them with opened pores from the warm water. If you take a tub bath for pleasure, make sure you shower immediately after the bath!

CHAPTER 9

BREATHE IN FRESH AIR 24 HOURS A DAY

We need oxygen to help every cell of our bodies. Fresh air contains ozonated gases that cleanse the blood and nourish the brain. We spend way too much time indoors breathing indoor stale air. In times past, the primitive and natural material make up of homes allowed much more fresh air to enter the homes than now. We also have many man made materials in our homes that diffuse toxic gases into our environments. The snug construction of our homes ALSO allows the same air to be recycled many times with its airborne pathogens and chemicals being evenly, but harmfully, distributed throughout the home.

Getting outside, exercising, and breathing in large quantities of fresh air is essential for good health. Opening windows to let in fresh air 24 HOURS A DAY is necessary. Even when it is very cold, some fresh air needs to be available. Most air conditioning systems do introduce fresh air at all times. But most heating systems do not.

If you are in an environment where you can not get fresh air, an air purifier that releases positive and negative ions and even some very low concentrations of ozone will dramatically improve your air quality. Ecoquest is one of many companies that sell these valuable machines.

CHAPTER 10

REMOVE HOUSEHOLD PETS FROM YOUR LIVING SPACE

This subject is a very delicate one. I love watching animal behavior. It is one of the great wonders of the Creation. But, the scientific fact is that your pet may be making you sick. VERY SICK AS A MATTER OF FACT! Animals were meant to live outside, not sharing a living space with you, a human. They carry all sorts of parasites and microbes that, when kept indoors or allowed to occasionally go outdoors, pick up microbes to transfer to you, your furniture, your countertops, your rugs, your pillows, your sheets, your wash cloths, etc. Find your pet a good home or farm OR permanently let them live outside your home. Love people, not pets.

There are whole books and researches by Dr. Hulda Clark and others who prove your pets can make you VERY sick. There is proof that the parasites your pets carry can be transferred to you. Some of these parasites are causing some of our most deadly diseases. This is a modern and very serious issue that has to be addressed if a person wants to get well permanently.

I know of people who have died because they were not willing to give up the pets that were making them sick. Their efforts to get well were constantly being thwarted by the REINFECTION they were getting from their pets. They knew it, but would not give up their pets. These died too young and unnecessarily.

Let your pets live outside your home where they belong.

Breathing in one egg of certain parasites on a piece of pet hair can cause you to have diseases such as diabetes, asthma, and others.

Every person I have known personally who has died of leukemia or has had true asthma has had cats that freely roamed their homes. They have been allowed to go anywhere they pleased including the beds and countertops. A report in USA TODAY in January 2011 told that indoor pets can make you very ill.

Biblically unclean animals (Leviticus 11 and Deuteronomy14) carry more pathogens than Biblically clean animals. Their very nature as scavengers and predators has them eat dead, rotting, and decaying matter, (or other unclean animals) whether it is vegetable or animal. They encapsulate these pathogens in their bodies in order to isolate those pathogens from humans. That is their purpose in creation! They are the roaming garbage collectors of the earth. Now do you see how harmful to your health it is to keep them in your closed living space? Do you see how their licking your face, mouth, and hands can be harmful?

I read an article years ago that stated that you could get a parasite infection just from your dog licking your leg! The researcher had proven this as the site of the entry of the parasite was where the dog licked the patient!

If you love yourself and your family, the best place for your pet is outside your living space. You may not understand the ENORMITY of the impact on your health your pet can have because of your emotional attachment to your pet, but if you truly think they love you, then I know they would tell you...let me go outside so I do not make you sick and you can live to feed me many more years!

CHAPTER 11

GET RID OF YOUR PARASITES – KILL THEM AND ELIMINATE THEM

How do you tell someone who showers every day, washes his hands somewhat frequently, has his clothes laundered or dry cleaned regularly, wears clean underwear every day and thinks he is a fairly clean person in general that he probably has parasites? And that harboring these parasites are robbing him of what little nutrition he is getting out of the nutritionally defunct food he is eating!!

We all have parasites from the day we are born. There are little parasites that live at the base of our eyelashes on the day we are born. There are parasites that can go across the placenta from mother to child!

But, then, there are the ravaging parasites that can invade us and rob us of the nutrition that was intended for OUR cells and not their cells. There are sugar craving parasites and meat craving parasites and heavy oil craving parasites and dairy craving parasites. And there are parasites that are the actual cause of some of our most puzzling diseases. These are the parasites about which we need to be concerned.

It is absolutely a waste of time and money to start taking varied supplements to restore your health without first taking a thorough parasite cleanse. If you are basically healthy, drinking carrot/parsley juice and taking an herbal parasite cleanse formula such as Parathunder OR Pure Planet parasite cleanse along with neem capsules for at least a month at first and then 2 times a year for a week each will ensure continuing and better health.

Our ancestors took parasite cleanses yearly. In Europe today, most doctors prescribe "worming" medicine to their patients 2 times a year. Our forefathers in the USA would take castor oil, wormwood tea, garlic and onions, cod liver oil, a tea of green black walnut hulls, eat pumpkin seeds, even kerosene! and many other natural items to rid themselves of "worms." We basically have completely stopped that practice and need to re-establish it once again!

An interesting fact is that ALL the foods the children of Israel called for on their wilderness journey had anti-parasite qualities! Cucumbers, melons, leeks, onions, and garlic! Numbers 11:5

Another interesting fact is that pomegranate, the fruit on the hem of the high priest's garment as he served in the tabernacle and temple in Scripture, is a very strong, yet delicious, parasite killer in the digestive tract! Exodus 28:34

HOW DO WE, AS BASICALLY WASHED AND CLEAN INDIVIDUALS, GET PARASITES?

Have you ever eaten an unwashed fruit or vegetable? Even if produce is grown organically, there are naturally occurring parasites that thrive in soil and seek out succulent fruits and vegetables as their food sources. There are also airborne parasites that land on produce at any time.

Have you ever eaten at a restaurant? Although the US government, states, counties, cities, and towns have operating cleanliness procedures for public food establishments, the individual cleanliness of each restaurant is monitored by the management on a day-to-day basis. There are parasites that are not even killed by 180 or 200 degree washing temperatures. And think about how many people have eaten off that heavy silver fork and creamy dinnerware and the different types of meat that have been on it.

Have you ever eaten at a fast food restaurant where an immigrant is assembling or handing you your food? In times long past, legal immigrants were made to stay on islands in New York City and San Francisco isolated for a period of time to see if they were bringing any diseases into the country. Today, legal immigrants are not thoroughly checked and tested for the many diseases and parasites rampant in foreign countries, let alone illegal immigrants who are flooding our country. It is not that they are purposely infected or purposely want to infect us, but we must understand that many cultures outside of ours do not stress hygiene as we do in the USA even in elementary schooling. Coming from more humble and primitive surroundings, they can harbor parasites, bringing them to our country.

Have you ever touched a toilet seat in a public place and not washed your hands afterward?

Have you ever eaten pork? Trichinae can withstand extremely high temperatures without dying.

Have you ever eaten raw sushi?

Have you ever eaten any cooked meat except that which was thoroughly well done? Scripturally defined unclean flesh hosts many more parasites than Scripturally defined clean flesh by the very nature of these animals being scavengers. But even Scripturally defined clean flesh can have parasites dwelling in it if the surroundings are unsanitary and if the live animals are not treated regularly for parasites and if all of the flesh is not cooked at high enough temperatures for long enough time periods.

Have you ever walked barefooted? Hookworms and other parasites can enter through the dirt that touches the bottom of your feet.

Have you ever touched a grocery cart handle? Although you like to think everyone is as clean as you are and as your Mother taught you to be, it just is not so! As a rabbi told us as he was preparing to circumcise one of our church member's sons, the hardest thing to teach people is not Scriptural Hebrew or verb declensions, but to wash their hands!!

Have you ever touched a public door handle?

Have you ever changed a baby's diaper and not washed your hands afterward?

Have you ever let a pet live inside your home? Or have you sat on furniture in someone's home that allows pets inside? As I will show you later, all you need is one cat hair with one parasite egg on it to infect yourself to contract asthma or diabetes.

Have you ever touched a pet or farm animal and not washed your hands immediately?

Or kissed a pet or allowed a pet to lick your face or hands?

Have you ever kissed anyone on the lips?

Have you ever traveled outside of the USA?

Have you ever eaten outside of the USA?

Have you ever sat on the furniture in a home where there is a cat or dog or bird living in the home?

Have you ever breathed in a home where there is cat hair in the air or a bird in a cage?

Have you ever had sexual relations with anyone?

Have you ever had sexual relations with a man who was uncircumcised? Uncircumcised penises harbor many more pathogens than circumcised penises.

It was the spring and fall habit of mothers and grandmothers in families of the past to make sure all members were "wormed". In Europe, most doctors prescribe worm killing drugs twice a year, but it is not practiced in this country.

We know now there are over 200 different types of parasites that can possibly inhabit the human body. Some think there are even MORE. The USDA checks for very few parasites in foods and meats. It is just your responsibility to rid them from your body on a regular basis if you want full health.

HOW DO YOU KNOW IF YOU HAVE PARASITES?

Sometimes you do not know for sure.

Concerning the 200 plus types of parasites that can inhabit the human body, there are tests to determine if and how many types of parasites you have that will cost you thousands of dollars to run. But there are some signs that could indicate you have parasites.

You can sometimes see them passed in your stool. You can have wrongly diagnosed arthritis, chronic fatigue, fibromyalgia, and different bowel conditions, foul smelling stools, itching anus, patches of small raised bumps on arms or legs, deep itching in the ears, dry itching in the nostrils, foul smelling breath, muscle aches, hard lumps just under the skin or in the muscle, eating a lot and not gaining weight, having a tremendous appetite at all times and gaining weight, yet still feeling hungry, having constant cravings for meat, dairy, heavy oils, or sweets, and experiencing a crawling feeling in your anus, feeling a twitch in the same place at various times, feeling a pinching in the same area of your intestines from time to time, stomach or intestine growlings or "squeaks", grinding of teeth at night, frequent nausea, feeling a movement in the intestines without expelling gas, feeling a dullness or fullness anywhere in the digestive tract, sounds in your stomach like a small cat mewing, bags under the eyes, puffy skin over the eyes, "bowel sounds", small patches of red bumps on the skin are all also possible indications of the presence of parasites. All of these conditions can point to parasite infestation.

In the 1990's, Dr. Hulda Clark discovered that many conditions, for which conventional medicine can find no cure, yield their symptoms easily when treated as parasite and chemical pollutant combination caused. Some of these conditions are consistently found to be a certain combination of a certain microbe or parasite and a certain accompanying chemical pollutant. Many of these conditions that can be treated quickly, easily, painlessly, and non-invasively are AIDS, cancer, diabetes, asthma, muscular dystrophy, fibromyalgia, epilepsy, some bowel conditions, chronic fatigue, and muscle wasting diseases, arthritis, migraine headaches, and others. She also has discovered that some parasites produce bacteria and viruses in the human body that maintain and cause to prolong certain diseases and conditions. Some of my regimens for my clients are based on her and other researcher's findings.

If you have parasites and until you get rid of the parasites, it does not matter what quality and how nutritionally packed the food is you are consuming because the parasites will get a percentage of that food. And the more parasites you have, the greater percentage they are going to use! As a matter of fact, some people get WORSE on very adequate nutritional programs because of this fact- they are very adequately feeding the very parasites causing their health problem!

If you have parasites, they get the best of any food or supplement you consume. The more parasites and the more varieties of parasites you have, the less food and nutrients you consume actually gets to YOUR cells. So, in reality, having parasites can either starve you to death OR cause you great cravings and unchecked obesity. Why the two opposites?

In one case, the parasites can eat nearly everything you consume and leave you weak and depressed even though you KNOW you have eaten enough calories for your healthy body weight. Certain other parasites will cause you to have cravings because they are consuming only certain trace minerals or certain portions of foods that you are not getting, but leaving the calories for you to pack on as stored fat. It leaves you craving more food, even though you have eaten more than enough varied source calories for your desired healthy body weight. More on this in a later chapter on obesity and weight loss.

Because of this fact that most people have NEVER taken a thorough parasite cleanse, I urge everyone to take a comprehensive parasite cleanse at the very onset of every health building regimen I design for a 3 week to 3 month time period if possible and at least 2 times a year for at least 1 week each time thereafter. Parathunder or Pure Planet parasite cleanse and neem capsules coupled together are the best for this parasite cleanse.

When parasites die in the human body, they release all of their stored and manufactured viruses and bacteria. For this reason, I urge all of my clients to take strong, natural anti-bacterials and strong, natural anti-virals AT THE SAME TIME they begin a parasite-cleansing program. To fail to do this may bring on multiple bacterial and viral infections making you sicker than when you began and maybe sicker than you have ever been in your whole life!! I know of people who have taken parasite cleansing herbs without the antiviral and anti bacterial herbs who got very serious bacterial and viral infections from the die-off. Buried Treasure ACF and Herbal Healer Academy 500 Parts per Million Colloidal Silver, Penn Herb Golden Seal/Myrrh capsules, and Kyolic Odorless Garlic#100 capsules or caplets are some supplements used for this viral and bacterial cleanse.

The next chapter tells you how important it is to kill your parasites before you do ANY OTHER natural treatment.

CHAPTER 12

KILL PARASITES FIRST BEFORE ANY OTHER TREATMENT!!!!!

Get Rid of Parasites First

The very first thing you must do to get better health is rid your body of parasites. You can do hundreds of things to try to get better health, but until you rid your body of any parasites, you will not be able to totally regain your health. You can buy hundreds of dollar's worth of supplements and take them, but any parasites you have will get the greatest percentage of these supplements' nutrients. You will literally waste time and money on these supplements if you do not rid your system of the parasites first. I know of many clients who started nutritionally building themselves up without killing the parasites first WHO ONLY GOT WORSE BECAUSE THEY WERE VERY ADEQUATELY FEEDING THE VERY PARASITES CAUSING THEIR CONDITION!!! There are so many conditions that are the result of having parasites alone or in combination with bacteria, viruses, molds, fungi, or chemical pollutants, that you simply can not ignore them and allow them to continue living in your body.

In Europe and Asia, nearly every doctor prescribes a parasite cleanse to his patients 2 times a year. It is similar to our getting our teeth checked in the USA 2 times a year. Everyone does it routinely. Our ancestors took castor oil once or twice a year or ate wild onions frequently or ate bitter herbs once or twice a year to accomplish this. But in the last 50 to 75 years, we have completely stopped this practice much to our detriment.

Now we are exposed to a greater number of varieties of parasites because we get our food from worldwide sources instead of just local sources. Our food is picked and prepared at restaurants by unchecked (health wise) immigrants. A tremendous rise in international travel and eating can also spread parasites very quickly.

Because some of the major diseases are now known to be associated with a particular parasite, this is just another reason why getting rid of parasites first is a wise action. Cancer, AIDS, asthma, diabetes, some thyroid conditions, many bowel conditions, and many more health conditions are directly affected by very particular parasites. Cleansing these parasites brings about total recovery much faster.

The very most important reason you must get rid of parasites first is that some other pathogens quite often have a symbiotic relationship with the parasites. The parasite is usually the stronger partner in this relationship. Its presence maintains the life of the weaker partner. Therefore, you MUST kill the parasite first in order to eventually get rid of the weaker partner.

An example of this is HEP C infection. Hep C is a viral infection. My clients have had great success in completely overcoming Hep C by doing a parasite cleanse, then a viral and fungal cleanse afterward. Once the offending parasite, the stronger of the two partners, is gone, the virus is easier to eliminate. Possibly the parasite is PRODUCING the virus while alive. It is, in the least, protecting and nurturing its viability.

The best and most effective international parasite cleanse I have used with my clients is Parathunder (www.whitesagelanding.com) and Colonix (from www.drnatura.com) in combination with neem (www.allaboutneem.com) herb. This combination will kill over 200 types of parasites from all the continents. TYPICALLY, Parathunder should be taken from 7 to 21 capsules a day depending on how advanced the case is. Neem should be taken 1 or 2 capsules

1 to 3 times a day. A substitute for Parathunder is Pure Planet parasite cleanse.

Neem herb ALONE kills the parasite that causes Chagas disease, the most prevalent heart stopping disease in the world today.

As parasites die, they release their stored and manufactured bacteria and viruses. So if you take a parasite cleanse, it is IMPERATIVE you take an anti-viral and anti-bacterial formulas at the same time. If you do not, you may end up with the worst viral or bacterial infection or multiple infections you have ever had! Several people I know had this very thing happen to them. The best formula to take is BURIED TREASURE ACF and HERBAL HEALER ACADEMY 500 PARTS PER MILLION COLLOIDAL SILVER. BT ACF should be taken 1 tablespoon 3 times a day. HHA CS 500 PPM should be taken 1/2 teaspoon 3 times a day.

If you can not get this parasite cleansing formula or these anti-virals or anti-bacterials, you should get a formula that contains colloidal silver, myrrh, garlic, goldenseal, neem, pumpkin seed, fennel, wormwood, green black walnut hulls and cloves AT THE VERY LEAST.

The regimen of these things should be taken AT FIRST for 3 weeks. If ANY of the following results appear, continue taking them for at least 3 to 6 weeks.....or 7 days after the last appearance of any of these things after the first 3 weeks.

1.   A crawling feeling anywhere in your body from 24 hours to one week of your first dosage. It is the live and greatly disturbed parasites on the move.
2.   A feeling of parasites moving up your throat, out of your lungs to your throat, or in or out of your bowels or vagina.

3.   Vibrations in your digestive tract especially in your anus area, bowel noises you have never heard before, pinching feelings in the bowel, foul smelling stool, foul smelling urine, foul smelling intestinal gas, foul smelling burps, stool smelling like a smell you have never smelled before, the smell of rotting flesh in your nose or throat.

4.   The actual appearance of dead parasites in your stool in the toilet (take a picture or no one will believe you!). Look them up on the Internet under "parasite images". Common ones are bluish white, grayish white, or yellowish white long (many inches to many feet) worms that look like flattened pasta (tapeworms), reddish brown long worms that are about the diameter and length of a pick-up stick, flukes with a somewhat bell shape, cancer/fungal fuzzies that look like koosh balls (about the size of bouncy balls that come out of the gumball machines), small white rice size pin worms, and more.

5.   Vague pains or cramping in your long muscles (such as your arm or leg muscles).

6.   Finally feeling you have completely evacuated your bowels for the first time in a very long time.

When the parasites are finally dead and eliminated from your body, you will feel finally at peace with your body. You may not feel strong, but you will know from the calmness in your digestive tract, the loss of pain in your joints, the rise in your energy level, and the lack of a battle going on in your body. For some people it takes just one week on the parasite herbs. But for some it takes 3 weeks to 3 months to completely rid their body of everything living in there. This time period should cover all the life stages of all the possible parasites that can possibly inhabit the human body.

If you have a basically normal size body in every area except your tummy or stomach (your arms and legs are not fat), you very likely have parasites, need colon cleansing, and have gotten this stomach from the consumption of too many refined carbohydrates (cakes, cookies, soda, pies, ice cream or beer, etc). The herbs and a high percentage raw diet will bring the stomach back down to size in just a few weeks of diligent care.

If you have never had really good bowel function (a stool about 1 to 2 feet long, about 1 to 2 inches in diameter, light brown in color, very little smell to it, 2 or 3 times a day), then you may benefit by also taking a bowel cleanser at the same time you take the parasite program. COLONIX is the best colon cleanser my clients have used in conjunction with a parasite cleanse. It is a gentle, non-cramping, slow transit bowel cleanser. It has no laxative effects (no rapid transit that causes a loose stool or diarrhea, muscle weakening effect, electrolyte loss, and cramping). It only gently inflates and scrapes the lining of the intestines to fully blossom the intestines to remove possibly years' worth of accumulated and hidden waste. Several of my clients have lost up to 40 pounds!!!!!!!! of weight while on the parasite/viral/bacterial/intestinal waste program!!!! One scoop of Colonix once or twice a day is sufficient.

While doing any cleanse, it is equally important to start from this day forward ONLY PUTTING IN YOUR BODY THOSE FOODS THAT BUILD THE BODY. This would include only organically grown foods, ample fresh water, lots of fresh fruits and vegetables, and little or no sugar, chemicals, sodas, junk, junk, junk and worthless so-called foods. Live foods have life in them. Cooked foods have lost all their enzyme activity that transfers life to the cells. To rebuild your health, you have to eat much more raw food and fresh juices than cooked food to provide the repair factors and life factors and youth factors. Look at everything you put in your mouth and ask, "Is this going to do some good or harm to my body if I eat it?" It will revolutionize your eating habits and health if you will do this!

CHAPTER 13

ELIMINATE VIRUSES, BACTERIA, MOLDS, AND FUNGI

Parasites inside your body can produce and harbor their own viruses and bacteria. As they go through their life cycles, they release these viruses and bacteria into your body as individuals die. As long as certain parasites are inside your body, you could have a long standing bacterial or viral infection that just does not go away or respond to conventional treatment or it comes back periodically. This is because as long as the parasites are there, they will continually be producing and releasing these 2 types of microbes. You have to kill and eliminate the parasites FIRST and THEN work on destroying the viruses and bacteria they release as they die, disintegrate, and are eliminated by your body.

Parasites, viruses, fungi, molds, bacteria, and certain chemicals can also have a symbiotic relationship with each other. Some are kept active by being in an atmosphere of multiple chemical pollutants. A parasite may live symbiotically with a fungus producing a long standing fungal infection that just does not respond to treatment. If you kill the parasite FIRST, then you will be able to kill the fungus NEXT and permanently. You could have a mold infection that is being kept alive by its symbiotic relationship with a virus or bacteria. There are so many possible combinations of these pathogens that are producing so many modern, previously unheard of diseases that each stage has to be addressed in order to get complete healing in some cases.

I have found the most successful pattern of treatment is to kill-
parasites first,
then viruses and bacteria,
then fungi and molds,

then do a heavy metal cleanse.

By following this order, the hosts or stronger partners in the symbiotic relationships are killed first making it easier to kill the remaining weaker, dependent partners.

Most often, I urge my clients to take parasite killing herbs, virus killing herbs and bacteria killing herbs all at the same time. This eliminates a lot of the discomfort of die-off when the dying parasites release their manufactured, stored or symbiotic viruses and bacteria. They can continue to take the bacteria and virus killing herbs for a period of time after the parasite cleanse is done to kill off remaining viruses or bacteria.

CHAPTER 14

USE COMPREHENSIVE DIGESTIVE ENZYMES

In order for your cells to be repaired and fed, each cell must receive the nutrients. This seems to be very logical, but to achieve it is like running an obstacle course. There are certain goals that must be achieved before the next goal can proceed. The failure of EVEN ONE of these steps can cause a failure to heal and rebuild.

In my discovery that there are several things that work together that almost always bring about excellent health, the use of enzyme therapy came to be one of the main healing factors. Once you get rid of the parasites, now you are ready to get ALL the nutrients you take in digested and on their way to the cells. This is not as easy a task as it seems.

Enzymes digest or break down the whole foods into their smallest components to be reassembled by the cells for their individual tasks.

There are many things that decrease your ability to make your own enzymes. Stress, lack of protein, parasites, many drugs, use of bicarbonate of soda that stops digestion, POLLUTANT CHEMICALS, AGRICULTURAL CHEMICALS, extreme illness, stress on the immune system, and LACK OF ENZYMES all contribute to this. The most troubling of these factors is lack of enzymes because IT TAKES ENZYMES TO MAKE ENZYMES!!! As you find yourself under any of these body-stressing conditions, your body makes fewer enzymes. The fewer the enzymes you make, the less food you digest, and still fewer nutrients get to your cells and the fewer enzymes you make. It is a continual downward spiral until you semi-starve yourself into a degenerative condition.

But the good news is that if you take a comprehensive digestive enzyme with your food for a period of 3 to 6 weeks and eat adequate protein during this time, you build up your own body's ability to make its own enzymes. A comprehensive enzyme contains every single digestive enzyme your body makes at every step of digestion. Taking these enzymes with your food for a period of time fools your body into thinking all the enzymes are being produced, and you get complete digestion of your food. They digest completely the protein in your food and make these proteins available to start making your own enzymes.

For these reasons, I strongly urge everyone to take a comprehensive digestive enzyme for at least a 3 weeks' period while parasites are cleansed. These should be taken at every major meal for this time period.

One or two tablespoons of apple cider vinegar are a good substitute for hydrochloric acid in the stomach when it is not being produced sufficiently. If your stomach hurts or you have a lot of distress after eating, you may not be producing enough hydrochloric acid. You can do a simple test on yourself that will reveal if you are producing enough or too much. Put 1 tablespoon apple cider vinegar in an ounce of water. Drink this with every major meal. If the distress stops, you are NOT producing enough hydrochloric acid on your own. If it still hurts or is worse, you are over producing hydrochloric acid on your own. STOP THE APPLE CIDER VINEGAR if this is the case.

If you found out you are NOT producing enough hydrochloric acid, you can continue to take the apple cider vinegar for a week or two at every major meal and eat adequate protein at every meal, and soon you will be producing enough on your own.

If you are not making enough hydrochloric acid or other digestive enzymes, parasites and other microbes can live longer, more comfortably, and multiply unchecked in your body, also.

Garden of Life Raw Enzymes is a very good comprehensive digestive enzyme formula.

I have also found that some clients with bowel conditions seem to progress faster in colon cleansing when taking comprehensive digestive enzymes. It seems the enzymes help to fully digest and release some of the undigested materials accumulated over time in the length of the intestines. This sometimes results in a large weight loss in the abdominal area.

CHAPTER 15

INCREASE BOWEL CLEANSING AND ABSORPTION

If the parasites are gone and you are not sharing your food with them, and if your food is now being able to be broken down into its usable components, now we have to actually get the nutrients to the cells. Again, this sounds easy, but it is a formidable task.

The subject we are about to talk about is not dinner subject matter, and yet it is a VERY VITAL SUBJECT THAT MUST BE DISCUSSED AND ACTED UPON in order to achieve health. It is equally as important as parasite cleansing, the use of enzymes, the use of organically grown food, and the yet to be discussed issue of the use of green foods and probiotics. If this issue is not addressed, all the money and time spent in the purchase and preparation of the foods and supplements is completely wasted.

Every cell, every tissue, every organ, and every chemical reaction within the body receives its raw materials through the delivery system of the intestines and circulatory system. As the properly digested food mass passes through the intestines, small particles of nutrients pass through the intestinal wall to be picked up by the bloodstream to be carried to each and every individual cell. If the interior walls of the intestine are clean and alive, this process proceeds unhindered. But, in those countries where a typical Western or American diet is eaten, we have another one of those obstacles.

Let us liken our intestines to a long garden soaking water hose that has small holes along the sides. When the water flows, gentle streams of water should seep out of the hose. In like manner, if there is nothing coating the intestines, the nutrients can flow on to the bloodstream. Now let us liken what the typical

American diet leaves in the intestines as superglue. This superglue is smeared thick and completely on the walls of the intestines like a hose full of cement.

The diet of white flour, white sugar, greasy fried foods, and very little exercise to giggle it off, and very few fiber foods to scrape it off, forms and maintains this superglue. Not only that, this continual diet and lifestyle forms pockets of unmoved foods that can stay in the intestines for literally YEARS, making perfect homes and foods for bacteria and parasites.

In order for the digested food to pass over this intestinal wall to get to the bloodstream and cells, the wall must be clean. We have to dissolve and gently scrape down and out this superglue substance and prevent it from forming again. Eating all natural, whole organic foods (raw spinach is nearly a specific for this job) is the first step in this process, but doing that alone could take months to completely clear the intestine and reshape and rebuild the intestines for full absorption of nutrients.

When you are chronically and/or critically ill, and action to reverse a condition must be rapid, an intestinal cleanser and, in some cases, intestinal rebuilder, must be used to quickly, but not too violently or rapidly, clear the superglue substance. A fiber product usually containing the superior form of fiber found in flaxseeds does this. One excellent product is Colonix. Another is plain ground flaxseeds.

You DO NOT want to take any colon cleansing product combination that includes LARGE quantities of senna or cascara sagrada. These two herbs only rapidly flush out all the loose stool and lots of valuable water and electrolytes and do not flush out the super gluey substance we are trying to eliminate. You DO NOT want a laxative that rushes through the intestine. All you need is a gentle fiber and herb combination that has a slow, but steady, transit time in the bowel. This type of colon cleanser and rebuilder will gently and painlessly clean and reform the colon without distress to you.

The fiber product absorbs water in the intestine thereby slightly inflating the intestine. As this fiber SLOWLY passes through the intestine, it gently restores the original shape of the intestine as well as gently scrapes the wall of the super gluey, mucous coating. Because sometimes the intestine shrinks down to a very small diameter, and because of stress and poor eating habits, some people, BUT NOT ALL, experience a little discomfort the first few days of using a fiber product. It is important to persevere in the use of the fiber and to realize it is just doing its cleansing and refurbishing job. Massaging the area of the discomfort often helps push the fiber along on its way. Using heat and drinking extra fluids such as catnip or peppermint tea at this time may also help the discomfort. The fiber will also start cleaning out any pockets that may have formed and elasticity will begin to return as you continue on a full regimen to take you back to full health.

You will begin having larger, softer, more frequent bowel movements that will leave you with a more relaxed feeling. For some people, this starts within the first 24 hours. For others it could take up to 5 to 10 days before they notice a big difference.

This fiber should be taken as far away in time from the taking of your supplements as possible, so the nutrients in the supplements are not soaked up by the porous fiber.

My favorite colon cleanser and rebuilder product is Colonix at www.drnatura.com. Some clients progress faster in complete colon cleansing if they pair the colon cleanser with comprehensive digestive enzymes such as are in Garden of Life Raw Enzymes. These enzymes help digest and dissolve some of the undigested food in the intestines.

CHAPTER 16

MAYBE USE COLONICS

Some patients are so blocked up in their intestines that one to four colonics may be necessary to open up a large enough passageway for any quantity of stool to pass. It may also be necessary to use the colonics to empty the bowel to start healing. A colonic is a very high enema. The bowel is inflated with water, or a combination of herb tea and aloe vera juice from sources like Aloe1. Immediately drinking a multi-form probiotic drink like organic kefir or Garden of Life Raw Probiotics will insure the reintroduction of many forms of probiotics. The bowel flushes itself with the extra water.

Immediately following the last colonic, a 10 to 35 form acidophilus/bifidus formula should be taken daily for about 2 weeks to re-establish any or all of the beneficial bacteria washed out in the colonics. Garden of Life Raw Probiotics for Women Vaginal Care (men can take this,too)has 38 forms of probiotivcs- perfect for this purpose. Not all patients need colonics, but some will progress much faster, even to the saving of their lives if time is short, if they start with the colonics. Jethro Kloss saved many nearly dead people using this life saving procedure!

I suggest colonics for some health problems specifically in the bowel, but am very careful not to suggest them for EVERY health concern. It is always preferable to let the bowel heal itself if possible and not to disturb the flora(probiotics) of the colon. It is nearly always better to build on the flora that is already there. Nevertheless, SOME people will not progress fast enough unless colonics are used.

CHAPTER 17

RE-ESTABLISH ALL THE BENEFICIAL INTESTINAL BACTERIA STRAINS

Now that you have cleansed the bowel and rid it and your other organs of parasites, you need to make sure you have once again the beneficial bacteria in your intestines that you were born with. These bacteria (UP TO 300 DIFFERENT BENEFICIAL STRAINS!) have been part of your defense system from the day you were born into this microbe-laden environment. Your mother's breast milk contained most of these probiotics. Many chemicals put on foods, conventional medicine antibiotics, conventional drugs, frequent enemas, parasites, and frequent use of laxatives, conventionally grown meats, dairy, and eggs that are highly treated with many forms of antibiotics, even a single bout of diarrhea can wipe out the colonies of good bacteria that should always be growing in your intestines. These good bacteria destroy harmful bacteria and harmful chemicals that pass through the digestive tract so they do not get absorbed by the blood stream.

Have you ever noticed after taking a round of conventional antibiotics that your energy is completely wiped out for a few days? This is because the antibiotic kills off ALL bacteria in your system, including the beneficial ones (although there are some more specific conventional antibiotics now than in years past that only target very specific harmful bacteria). The good bacteria manufacture the energy producing B-complex vitamins in your body. Without these Bcomplex vitamins you feel weak, energyless, and limp. Once these particular strains of probiotics are re-established in your intestines, B complex production returns, and sufficient energy returns.

These bacteria can be replaced to a degree by eating organic yogurt and kefir (soy, coconut, or goat based to those who can tolerate them well), and comprehensive probiotics supplements like Garden of Life Raw Probiotics. At the writing of this book, several hundred different strains of beneficial bacteria have been found to inhabit the human intestine, doing protective jobs for the body. The supplement with the most strains now available (at the writing of this book) commercially is Raw Probiotics by Garden of Life Vaginal Care. It contains 38 OF THE MOST STUDIED AND PROVEN HEALTH PROTECTING strains of beneficial probiotic bacteria. Yes, men can take this!

A reminder- when looking for a comprehensive probiotic, look for the one with the most individual strains of probiotics. The "millions and billions" numbers mean very little compared to how many individual acidophilus and bifidus strains are present.

Make sure the supplement you buy has MANY forms of probiotics. My favorites are Raw Probiotics by Garden of Life (there are several varieties within this brand), Mega Foods Mega Flora, Flora Source, LB-17, and NSI 15-35. Eating bananas, carrots, goat, coconut, or soy kefir, and lactic acid foods help these bacteria to grow rapidly after having been reintroduced into your system.

Studies of cultures where a great proportion of the population of the people live to over 100 year old almost always consume a cultured dairy product DAILY. The constant daily replenishing of the beneficial bacteria ensure a healthy immune system against incoming pathogens.

CHAPTER 18

REMOVE MOUTH METAL

If you have dentist placed metal in your mouth, you will be swallowing small amounts of the dissolved metal as long as the metal is there. Some of the metals such as mercury, tin, lead, nickel, and isotopes, etc. used in metal fillings and dental work are highly toxic. There has been a great debate for many years over the decision to completely outlaw the use of these metals in dental amalgams. In every dentist's office there is a specifically marked and designated toxic metal disposal area for these fillings that have been removed from patient's mouths!

Some clients do not get complete healing from their condition (breast cancer is first on this list) until they have all of this metal removed from their mouths. For a complete discussion of this issue, the book, IT'S ALL IN YOUR HEAD, by Dr. Hal Huggins discusses the scientific findings in this area. Starting with your next visit with your dentist, you should ask that only white porcelain fillings be used in your mouth for new and replaced fillings. And, if you can afford it, you should have all the mouth metals of crowns, posts, bridges, etc. replaced with safe plastic or porcelain. If full dentures are needed, make them totally plastic.

Pockets of bacteria can be found sometimes under old or damaged fillings. Improperly treated root canals can also have these areas of infection called cavitations. It is good to have root canal pockets checked from time to time to see if they are breeding bacteria. An endodontist can do this for you.

Burdock root and cilantro remove these toxic metals mentioned above once the source is gone. One or two cups of burdock tea daily for 3 weeks and/or one fresh bunch of cilantro eaten daily for about 3 weeks accomplish ridding your body of these toxic chemicals.

CHAPTER 19

RID YOUR HOME OF ALL TOXIC CHEMICALS

There are literally hundreds of toxic solvent type chemicals that are in your home in the furniture, flooring, fabrics, plastic surfaces, and chemical cleaners you use to clean nearly everything. These solvents constantly "off-gas" solvent fumes into the air in your home. These solvents are products of the petro industry and soak into your tissues setting up a perfect environment for many unhealthy conditions to flourish. Take as many of these chemicals as you can out of the home and store them in an outside building not sharing a roof with your home. Replace them with natural cleaning items like apple cider vinegar, baking soda, grapefruit oil, orange oil, pine oil, lemon juice, etrog, peroxide, borax, diluted ammonia, etc. Storing the solvents outside your living space eliminates one very strong deterrent to accomplishing your complete healing.

If you are fortunate enough to be able to build a new home, try to make as many things in the home from natural sources and as health protecting as possible. Using wood, bamboo, glass, stone, ceramic tile, linen, cotton, hemp, seacell and other natural materials is healthier than using synthetic materials. Build in windows that actually open. A screen room or porch can be used as a sleeping room in temperate weather. Use hardwood floors and tile as much as possible throughout the home. A SMALL SINK OR FOUNTAIN JUST OUTSIDE THE MAIN DOORS CAN BE USED BY PEOPLE ENTERING YOUR HOME BEFORE THEY ACTUALLY BRING PATHOGENS INTO THE HOME. A entry way can be built to leave shoes in before entering the home. All natural fabrics like linen can be used for furniture coverings, drapes, and bed linens. The books THE NATURAL HOME and THE NATURAL HOUSE detail how to accomplish a home with nearly all all natural building materials and furnishings.

CHAPTER 20

TAKE A TOXIC HEAVY METAL AND CHEMICAL POLLUTANT CLEANSE

Once the metals are out of your mouth and home, a toxic metal cleanse can be taken. This is started by taking burdock root tea and a whole bunch of fresh chopped cilantro daily for at least 3 weeks. You can add to that Toxinout capsules or Daily Detox (black box) tea to complete the removal of toxic metals and other chemical pollutants.

CHAPTER 21

EAT A LOT OF GREEN FOODS

If you are eating a typical American or Western diet, I want you to think of how much green food you have had in the past week. Was it one leaf of yellowish lettuce on a hamburger?? Or a little cup of cabbage smothered in mayonnaise?

We need green food only second to protein. There are micro chemicals, vitamins, and minerals absolutely necessary to the continuation of life in green foods that cannot be found in ANY other type of food!!! The chlorophyll present in these foods sanitizes and disinfects the body, and we cannot live prosperously without just THAT ONE component of green foods. We need several cupfuls of fresh, RAW, untainted green foods and a healthy serving of a cooked green food EVERY DAY!!! Kale, collard greens, turnip greens, endive, rape, rapini, frisee, beet greens, broccoli, broccolini, parsley, lettuces, cabbages, cilantro, seaweeds or sea greens, or others should be eaten EVERY DAY.

Green foods were permitted and commanded in Genesis 9:3 as food for mankind.

Green foods bring valuable oxygen and fiber into the body. Oxygen kills certain pathogens on contact. And the fiber keeps things moving along in the intestines so toxic chemicals do not get absorbed by the intestine. Fiber also absorbs and encapsulates some toxic chemicals escorting them out of the body.

In some cases, where busy people have no time to do quality cooking, I advise them to take a dried or freeze dried organic green product to fill in this need on a daily basis. All my clients who are critically and chronically ill take a dried organic green product, whether it is wheat grass, alfalfa, spirulina, sea kelps, or dried barley, or a mixture of many of these dried greens or a fresh glass of greens' juice or several servings of chlorophyll liquid daily. Perfect Food by Garden of Life, Green Vibrance, Marine Greens, Reservage Organic Greens and Barley Max are some of my favorites. Mint flavored chlorophyll liquid could be taken every day for the rest of your life!

CHAPTER 22

TO EAT MEAT OR TO NOT EAT MEAT? WHERE TO GET COMPLETE PROTEIN

Many people ask me if I eat meat. I am mostly a vegan/fins and scales fish eater. I eat mostly green vegetables, fruits, root vegetables, beans, seeds, nuts sparingly, and small amounts of high protein grains. I try to stay dairy free and gluten free as much as possible (although I occasionally will eat a little when nothing else is available). I eat wild caught fish occasionally. I usually eat a little turkey each Thanksgiving. And I always eat organic lamb on Passover. Maybe once every few months I will eat green or grass fed beef, buffalo, or chicken. I can not lie. It is true. But most of the time...98% of the time...I eat vegan.

And most of the time about 80% of my vegan food is always raw, fresh, and ripe.

After reading the book MAD COWBOY by Howard Lyman, I REFUSE TO EAT COMMERCIALLY GROWN CONVENTIONAL BEEF OR CHICKEN. I URGE YOU TO READ THIS BOOK. You will not be able to recover your health unless you understand what is being done to our food supply including WHAT IS HAPPENING TO THE MEATS FOR THE LOVE OF MONEY. I feel the commercial meat supply is totally unsanitary at this point in time. Since the Father in Heaven made cows to eat only vegetable products and farmers are feeding them animal by-products, they have made carnivores, and possibly cannibals, out of herbivores, a very unnatural switch. To this add all the antibiotics they are fed, all the diseases that are passed around as individual animals from many farms are added to an already huge herd, all of the parasites that go unchecked and untreated in them, and all the growth hormones that are pumped into them. All of these negative, NON-FOOD things pass to us upon consumption of their flesh.

I believe the Father gave us permission to eat certain animals. They are referred to as "clean" animals or as kosher animals by the Jewish people, Messianic believers, and the Scriptures. These animals are browsing animals and not scavenger animals. If they had continued in their wild, free roaming state, they would still be good for us. If we could all hunt buffalo, moose, elk, etc. like is and was done in Alaska, the Northern and Western states, we could feel much better about the healthy state of our meat.

There are some very conscientious farmers who are trying to produce organically grown, grass fed, green fed, open air or small processor processed animals for meat. If you absolutely have to eat meat, patronize these farmers as they are trying to produce meat that is actually healthy for you. Grass fed meat has so many benefits over grain fed meat. THE MOVIE FOOD, INC. DELVES INTO THE IMPLICATIONS OF GRAIN FED ANIMALS ABOUT WHICH YOU SHOULD INFORM YOURSELF THOROUGHLY.

The animals in the conventional commercial meat industry that are called "clean" animals (in the reference to Scriptural law) are being manipulated for profit and not with our health in mind. We have the evidence they are being now made unsanitary and most likely unfit for human consumption.

However, you do need complete protein. Complete protein is a protein combination that provides all the 22 amino acids needed to build and repair body tissue and body function chemicals. All animal products have complete protein - meat, dairy, eggs, poultry, and fish. If you choose to not eat animal flesh and animals' by-products, your body still needs complete protein. There are several complete protein vegetable sources, so it is not necessary to eat meat as long as you get plenty of the vegetable sources of complete protein.

Here is a list of these vegetarian complete protein foods. They all have the 22 essential amino acids to rebuild body tissues.

Millet

Amaranth

Buckwheat

Hempseed

Quinoa

Spirulina

Hummus

Chia

In Africa, there are tribes who eat only millet and fruits. These people have nearly perfect health.

The following foods are ALMOST complete protein foods...

Potato

Broccoli

Lentils

Spinach

Most cultures have figured out by how they feel (full, satisfied, repairing, and growing!) after they eat certain combinations of foods which make complete protein. In the Middle East, they eat

a grain and a bean plus a seed

such as in falafels (wheat pocket breads plus garbanzo beans or chickpeas plus sesame seeds in the tahini). In South America, they eat beans plus a grain (corn tortillas and beans) or a

bean plus a seed (black beans and rice). In the Far East, they eat a

seed plus a bean (soybeans and rice). Chemical analysis reveals that

a bean plus a grain equals complete protein. Also a

bean plus a seed equals complete protein.

If you add either a grain, bean, or seed to these combinations, you add quality to the already existing complete combination. The book DIET FOR A SMALL PLANET BY Frances Moore Lappe written many years ago is still the bible of vegetarian protein combining.

CHAPTER 23

COW MILK, OTHER MILKS, AND DRINKS

85% of the world's population drinks goat milk. 85%! And most of these people do not have obesity problems. And most of them do not drink much goat milk once they are adults. Goat's milk is the closest in composition to human breast milk of any milk used around the world.

Cow's milk has THE FAT, PROTEIN, and HORMONE CONTENT to make a baby calf grow to a full grown cow within about a year or two. Cow's milk has the hormones to make a female cow grow huge udders to nurse one or two baby calves. Cow's milk has hormones to make a baby calf grow to a huge cow. Now do you see why you are so BIG?

Goat milk makes a slim baby goat grow into a slim adult goat. Goat milk has hormones and fats that make a slim baby goat grow into a SLIM adult goat. Most of the people in the world who rely on goat milk are slim.

Most commercial soy, almond, grain, hemp, oat, and rice milks have sugar in them to make the taste better. Sugar is sugar no matter where you get it. If you use any of these, get the plain, unsweetened kind .Even better yet is to make your own at home and add a little natural sweetener like dates or honey or stevia when blending.

There is machine named Soybella that makes soy, almond, and grain milks at home without added sugar. Blend-tec, Ninja 2500, and Vita-mix and other high powered super blenders are valuable to make you own milks, too.

There is so much that could be said against the drinking of cow milk. The book DON'T DRINK YOUR MILK by Frank Oski and the books MILK A—Z and MILK, THE DEADLY POISON by Robert Cohen will both make you want to never drink cow milk or cow milk products again. Arm yourself with the facts to help your daily decision making easier and more informed. Of course, some of these reasons to not drink cow's milk is because of the way the products are processed.

We should be demanding as consumers organic goat milk be available in gallon jugs as easily as cow's milk is now. Many other countries have it easily available!

If cows were raised with original methods, the meat and milk would be very good for us.

WHAT ELSE CAN I DRINK?

There is water, naturally flavored waters with no sugar added, water, flavored waters with no artificial sweeteners added, water, 100 % organic FRESH fruit and vegetable juices, water, grain coffees, water, herb teas (cold or hot), freshly made grain beverages (in a Soybella machine).

Remember when juice used to be served in those very small 3 or 4 ounce glasses? That is as much as you need at one time and only once or twice a day!

You might have notice I mentioned water quite a bit!! That is what you need more than anything else!

CHAPTER 24

GLUTEN AND BREAD YEAST

Many of the grains we use today are hybrids of the grains available in ancient times. On top of that, the white flour is laced with chemicals that are disturbing to the digestive system. Our constant consumption of the same food over and over and over again, especially of it is a half food (like white flour is) and contaminated with non-food chemicals, makes our body want to reject it over time. All of these facts add up to sometimes an intolerance of a certain class of foods, like gluten containing grains over time. These intolerances can end up finally manifested as the bowel and intestinal problems we see so prevalent today like Crohn's disease, ulcerative colitis, colitis, irritable bowel syndrome, etc.

However, some things thought to be gluten intolerance may actually be glyphosate poisoning or GMOs harming your body or the repeated use of the same baking yeast in the bread.

We do not absolutely need to have grains in our diet. We can get the starch (carbohydrates) and B vitamins and other trace minerals from fruits, beans, and dark green vegetables.

And there are grains that do not contain gluten, which are whole grains, which are welcome unique changes from the gluten containing grains.

- Gluten containing grains –

Wheat

Oats

Rye

Barley

Spelt

Kamut

- Non-gluten grains -

Corn

Rice

Quinoa

Gluten free oatmeal

Millet

Buckwheat

Chia (seed)

A factor that may get confused as a gluten intolerance is the presence of bread yeast. Some people, in truth, really have no trouble with gluten, but think they do when the offender is actually the bread yeast in the gluten containing bread. Again, the yeast used to make commercial bread is not exactly the same as a natural yeast found in sour dough (using an airborne starter). If you feel you might have a gluten intolerance, experiment with using a flatbread without yeast to see if it is better tolerated. Of course, you can eliminate both also to see if your health and digestion improve. If you end up going gluten free in your diet, also make sure that the other grains you do use are WHOLE GRAINS.

Another thing to consider about grains is if they are GMO or not. GMO - genetically modified organisms- are just that. The many foods including most grains that are not organic labeled have been modified genetically, and the body recognizes that and rejects them. Many of today's digestive problems are because of the use of GMOs in foods. Your only assurance you do not eat these is by buying organically grown grains and products marked organic

CHAPTER 25

USE COMPREHENSIVE, CONCENTRATED WHOLE ORGANIC FOOD SUPPLEMENTS

Using all the above-discussed aspects of building your health will eventually bring about a total cure. I have seen it happen too many times over 50 years to deny the truthfulness of the benefits of this way of living and eating. But I have been approached many times by people who are about dead from the effects of their faulty living who need a fix and need it fast. These cases have been the most initially frightening, challenging, and finally satisfying to me personally. I have felt I have been a bystander many times, watching a miracle take place in front of my eyes. We pray, we fast sometimes, and we load them up 24 hours a day with the most highly concentrated, full spectrum nutrient herbal supplements that they can handle. And they get better, and they get better very rapidly!!!

There has been wonderful research and documentation of the effects of individual nutrients on the body and its recuperative process over the past century. But I have found I get quicker and more complete results with a client if, instead of taking 10,000 mgs. of vitamin C a day alone, for example, a client takes, in addition to high dosages of individual highly depleted nutrients, several whole highly concentrated food products (individual herbs, Perfect Food, Green Vibrance, NutraRev by Peter Gilliam, VM100 by Buried Treasure, Natural Vitality Organic Life, Marine Greens, 6 Seaweed Formula by Naturespirit Herbs, etc.) which supply ALL of the systems small amounts of HUNDREDS of necessary nutrients at the same time. Adding to these concentrated products specific nutrients known to be missing in different conditions usually brings about rapid disappearance of symptoms.

The weakest usually say within a three-day period from commencing a concentrated regimen that they have never felt the life strength that they are feeling at this point!!! Whenever I see this happen and see the happiness and renewed hope in a client's voice and eyes, I remember sitting in my basic nutrition course at Cornell University. Our professor told us that if even one nutrient were missing in sufficient amounts, total health could not be achieved.

The regimens at the end of this book contain all the principles outlined above, combined into comprehensive, healing programs. The most effective elements of these regimens are the herbal combinations that are strong to make positive changes in your body without stressing the body.

CHAPTER 26

DO INDIVIDUAL ORGAN CLEANSES

Sometimes clients have so abused their bodies for years and they are so critically ill, when they start the cleansing and rebuilding process, their organs are totally overloaded with waste. These clients have to take time to clean these individual organs for the healing process to continue. Most of my clients take several liver flushes and a kidney cleanse sometime near the beginning of the regimen set up for them. These cleanses have been made widely popular by Dr. Hulda Clark, although many natural practitioners have urged their use for many years. Even athletes notice a great surge in their energy after these cleanses.

The one day liver flush outlined below can be done once every 3 weeks until you are well. This releases gall stones and any flakes or obstructions in the liver, hepatic duct, and gall bladder. The magnesium helps relax the tissues and the olive oil lubricates as the waste is eliminated.

ONE DAY SIMPLE LIVER FLUSH

THIS MAY BE DONE ONCE BEFORE STARTING A REGIMEN.

DONE 3 WEEKS APART STARTING AT DAY 21 UNTIL DAY 84 (4 DIFFERENT ONE DAY LIVER FLUSHES, EACH 3 WEEKS APART) CHILDREN MAY TAKE ½ OR ¼ DOSAGES ACCORDING TO WEIGHT AND AGE
CHOOSE A WEEKEND DAY TO DO THIS LIKE A FRIDAY NIGHT OR A SATURDAY NIGHT.

MIX TOGETHER—

3 CUPS WATER OR HOMEMADE FRESH HONEY LEMONADE
4 t. EPSOM SALTS (MAGNESIUM SOURCE)
½ CUP OLIVE OIL
2/3 CUP FRESHLY SQUEEZED PINK GRAPEFRUIT JUICE

MIX ALL TOGETHER AND DIVIDE INTO 4 JARS WITH LIDS. REFRIGERATE.

DO NOT EAT ANYTHING AFTER 4 PM.

AT 4 PM, 6 PM, 8 PM, AND 10 PM DRINK CONTENTS OF ONE JAR.
At 10 PM, ALSO TAKE 5 PARATHUNDER OR 1 TEASPOON PURE PLANET PARASITE CLEANSE.

GO TO BED WITH HEAD ELEVATED ON ONE OR TWO PILLOWS.

IF YOU WAKE UP IN THE NIGHT, DRINK LOTS OF WATER.

UPON ARISING, DRINK LOTS OF WATER.

YOUR FIRST BOWEL MOVEMENT OF THE DAY SHOULD BE SOFT, GREENISH, AND CONTAIN GALLSTONES AND OTHER LIVER TOXINS AND OTHER DEBRIS. IF NOTHING HAPPENS, IT WILL ON YOUR SECOND OR THIRD CLEANSE.

REPEAT IN 3 WEEKS AT 6 WEEKS, IN 9 WEEKS AND IN 12 WEEKS UNTIL YOU HAVE DONE A TOTAL OF 4 CLEANSES.

HERBAL KIDNEY CLEANSE

MIX TOGETHER EQUAL PARTS OF THE FOLLOWING DRIED HERBS-

GRAVEL ROOT

HYDRANGEA TROOT

MARSHMALLOW

UVA URSI

PARSLEY

PUT 1 HEAPING TABLESPOON OF HERB MIXTURE IN 1 CUP BOILING WATER. STEEP. DRINK 2 CUPS A DAY FOR ABOUT 3 WEEKS.

These herbs are already pre-mixed in the product by the Longevity Corporation named Kidney-Bladder Detox Tea.

In the next few chapters we will discuss some things that affect your health that are not necessarily nutrition oriented, but nonetheless affect your ability to get totally well. These non-nutritive factors must also be addressed to help you on your way to getting well.

CHAPTER 27

GET SOME MOVEMENT

No matter how weak or debilitated the patient is, movement is an accelerating factor in recovery. Even the smallest amount of movement can help digestion, increase the circulation, help the elimination of toxins and microbes, and even stimulate the appetite. The patient can just move in bed by raising arms, legs, or head, rock gently in a rocking chair, or sit and bounce gently on a mini-trampoline. As strength increases, more vigorous movement is possible. Even short walks contribute to rehabilitation from most conditions.

CHAPTER 28

GET DAILY SUNSHINE

All patients should spend 20-30 minutes a day in a protected area in the sun. Sunshine has powerful anti-depression and anti-microbe qualities.

This does NOT include the use of tanning beds. Tanning beds are very dangerous. Scientific evidence shows that even ONE visit to a tanning bed increases the likelihood of skin cancer by 4 times compared to those who have never used a tanning bed!!!!

Although some doctors have warned of our staying out of the sunlight to prevent skin cancer, I feel the opposite is true. Most people are getting LESS DAILY sunlight than their predecessors did and yet are still getting skin cancer. One PROOF that this is true is that most people have too little Vitamin D in their bodies.

But today we MAY be exposing way too much TOTAL SKIN AREA at a time (TOO FEW CLOTHES!) to the sun, even if for shorter periods of time. Getting in the sun produces Vitamin D, which prevents skin cancer and other health problems. If you get cancer after being in the sun, there were factors in your skin that would have produced skin cancer, eventually, whether you got in the sun or not.

It has been proven 100% linen clothing protects your skin the most from the sun, and it releases the most heat and moisture on a hot day. And yet it feels light on the body!

Propyl alcohol in any form is found in most cancers and most certainly skin cancer. This chemical is found in nearly every commercial personal care product we use on our bodies like shampoo, liquid soaps, hand lotion, aftershave, deodorant, skin creams, over the counter skin medicines, perfumes, etc. I will write more about this in a later chapter. Some other non-natural source chemicals even in sunscreen react adversely with sunlight, affecting our skin.

CHAPTER 29

SEEK PERFECT PEACE AND OBEDIENCE

There is nothing like being at perfect peace with yourself, your neighbor, and your Creator. This alone can restore health to a perfect condition by the miraculous power of the Creator. There are missionaries and POW's that have been denied all the above mentioned things that give health whose lives were maintained intact by just trusting the One Who knows them best and has promised to take care of them no matter what the circumstances. Take time to get acquainted with your Creator. Not doing this is like trying to run and fix a complicated piece of machinery without reading the instruction book. The Scriptures have all the answers to all the tough questions in life. As George W. Bush said when asked which philosopher most influenced his life, "Christ, because He changed my heart." This is the ONLY way you will get peace. When your heart is changed by the power of the Creator, peace floods every part of your body.

THE SPIRITUAL AFFECTS THE PHYSICAL AND THE PHYSICAL AFFECTS THE SPIRITUAL

As you learn more spiritually and physically, you will see what you do physically affects your spiritual blessings and what you do spiritually affects your physical blessings. Deuteronomy 27-30 teaches this plainly. Conventional medicine tries to box the physical and the spiritual separately, but the Scriptures speak of their intertwining constantly.

The Hebrew word for "faith" involves a greater scope than the meaning we have for it in English. Hebrew indicates "faith" as a thought process/belief system that leads to immediate obedience to the Creator's will and loving instructions.

The modern, evolved meaning leans toward a thought process of just believing in the Creator but not necessarily including acting in an immediate obedient manner.

Almost all of the Creator's blessings are conditional upon belief plus faith and belief- and faith-motivated action (obedience). He gives out some blessings and things to all, to believers and non-believers, like rain, sunshine, heat, cold, fresh air, food growing on the earth, the possibility of employment in the realm of worldly business for the benefit and service of other men. And sometimes He withholds even these basic blessings to awaken believer and non-believer to their wayward lifestyles.

There are other deeper and wider blessings He promises to them that have decided to follow all of His ways in every aspect of their lives. To these He promised a higher form of life or the highest form of life that can be lived in this life. One place in the Scripture He calls it riding on the high places of the earth (Isaiah 58). In great humility, I tell you as I have yielded myself to ALL of the Creator's commands, I have seen and experienced this life of fullness, abundance, protection under persecution, power, interventions, deliverances, gifts and wisdom of the Holy Spirit, the voice of leading and warning, dreams, visions, wonders, constant answers to prayers and fastings, CONSTANT PROVISION, AND LACK OF WANT. He absolutely promises these things and more IF WE BELIEVE AND IF WE OBEY THE DETAILS OF HIS WORD.

We have been told by many preachers this or that is not necessary any more to do that are written plainly in the Scriptures. You can believe them or you can believe Messiah who said,

"Think not I am come to destroy the law." (Matthew 5:17) and

"The scribes and Pharisees sit in Moses' seat. All therefore whatsoever they bid you observe, that observe and do" (Matthew 23:2-3) and

"Man shall not live by bread alone, but by EVERY WORD that proceeds out of the mouth of the Creator" (Matthew 4:4) and

"For whosoever shall keep the whole law and yet offend in one point, he is guilty of all" (James 2:10) and

"If you love me, keep my commandments" (John 14:15)

"Go, and sin no more" (John 8:11)

"Bring forth therefore works worthy of repentance" (show by your works that you are intending to stop disobeying the laws of the Creator) (Luke 3:8)

"That they should repent (stop sinning) and turn to the Creator, and do works meet for repentance (worthy of acknowledging wrong and initiating change)" (Acts 26:20)

"Sin is the transgression of the law" (1 John 3:4) and

"Do we make void the law through faith? Our Creator forbid: yea, we establish the law" (Romans 3:31)

"Shall we continue in sin that grace may abound? Our Creator forbid. How shall we that are dead to sin continue any longer therein?" (Romans 6:1, 2)

" Whosoever therefore shall break one of these least commandments, and shall teach men so, he shall be called the least in the kingdom of heaven: but whosoever shall do and teach them, the same shall be called great in the kingdom of heaven." (Matthew 5:19)

Once the Creator sets down a law, it is in force until He Himself says the law is not in effect. The laws about our health and spiritual life and physical life all affect our physical life and physical health.Messiah said all laws from the Creator will be in effect until heaven and earth pass... and as far as we can see, that has not happened YET!

Deuteronomy 27 through 30 lumps all of the Creator's laws under one banner. Messiah reiterated this in Matthew 4:4, Matthew 5:17, and Matthew 23:1, 2. James the apostle restated it in James 2:10. If you disobey any of them, you may have spiritual and/or physical cursing. Serving the Creator is a package deal with many aspects to it. It is easy to obey once you know what is expected of you. It can be compared to a new job description. Just as a new job may look hard when first approaching it, after you understand what is expected of you in the job description, you apply yourself to fulfill the job description and you receive a paycheck for doing the job for which you have been hired.

If you spend your days in sin, the wages you will receive is death. But if you apply yourself totally to Scripture as life guidelines, you will receive life, abundant life now and eternal life in the future, as your pay. Blessing and freedom from the curses promised to those who ignore, minimize, rebel against, shift to antiquity, or refuse to do the Creator's will and ways will be yours.

You can not have peace in the innermost of your being until you are at peace with your Creator. This only happens when you surrender all that is you to Him and His will. He has already set up for you the perfect way to live outlined in the Torah or His instructions for the best life possible in this life. All the good things that you desire in life are prepackaged in this life He has preplanned for you in His instructions. The way to peace is living within the beautiful confines of His will.

CHAPTER 30

GETTING READY AND GETTING STARTED

When someone comes to Natural Herbal Therapy for help, we start with a doctor's diagnosis. We must be satisfied that the client really knows exactly what is wrong with his health before he can start fixing it for the better. Usually he has very specific medical tests to determine what condition he has.

The client fills out a Client Worksheet asking him to reveal what he is experiencing head to toe. He states also what drugs, over the counter drugs, and natural supplements he has taken in the last few months and the reasons he was taking them. He also lists what vaccinations, immunizations, innoculations, and flu shots he has had.

After reading and evaluating all the information given on the Client Worksheet, an individualized regimen is designed for him with all natural suggestions for the client to address all of their health problems as quickly and efficiently as possible.

I do not heal anyone. The herbs, juices, teas, and natural supplements heal the person. The agents and their actions in the body in these supplements are known by many researches and publicly available publications. The clients are in full control of their own healing by the different supplements they allow to enter their body.

In general, with all clients, we start with a 3 week to a 3 month parasite cleanse with added natural antivirals and antibacterials. The client is strongly urged to eat only a vegan diet for this time period to avoid recontaminating himself with the same or other parasites during the parasite cleanse. Some continue this vegan diet for the rest of their lives. They are asked to remove any household pets from their environment before the parasite cleanse for at least the time of the parasite cleanse. Some give their pets away permanently.

The client usually starts a fiber product and a complete digestive enzyme formula, as well as a multiple form probiotic. At week 3, 6, 9, and 12, a one day liver flush is taken. After week 6 a kidney cleansing tea is added daily for a week. Also after week 6, any known nutrients that are deficient will be added to the diet temporarily to bring the levels back up to normal.

If his primary health problem is in the bowel, we might give him 1 to 4 colonics. These are ONLY used in the most desperate cases. It is more important to maintain and build on the present intestinal flora if at all possible. If colonics are given, I have them start taking a COMPREHENSIVE (at least 15 to 35 forms) probiotic formula such as Raw Probiotics by Garden of Life, Mega Foods Mega Flora (6 the first day and 2 to 3 every day thereafter) or NSI 15-35 immediately.

They are urged to rid their home of household pets and scavenger animals (Leviticus 11 and Deuteronomy 14), which will most certainly constantly and continually reinfect them. They are urged to remove or steam clean very thoroughly any upholstered furniture, bed linens, bath linens, or curtains that may have pet dander, hair, fur, feces, or urine on or in them. Some of my clients have felt their homes were so infiltrated with the filth of the animals they kept as pets that they have literally left their homes and started fresh with a new home and furnishings. Not everyone can do that, but some have in order to have every chance at rebuilding their health.

They are urged to use only glass cookware like white Corning ware or clear or colored Fire King. Even stainless steel cookware may leach nickel. Aluminum cookware is not acceptable anymore as a cooking surface because of its possible role in Alzheimer's disease. Aluminum forms flakes on foods as they are cooked in it that are then ingested.

They are urged to have a dental checkup and start removing silver colored fillings containing nickel, tin, and mercury, replacing them with white porcelain fillings.

They are urged to remove from their home any solvent type chemicals to an outside, unattached building.

They are asked to clean their heating and air conditioning systems.

They are urged to completely clean their homes, using pine and/or antibacterial cleaners.

They are urged to always take off their shoes before entering their homes so as not to bring any of the microbes of the outside environment into their homes.

They are urged to remove rugs and replace with easily cleaned hardwoods or tile, if possible.

All of these things are always easier to address upon moving to a new home, but if that is not possible, the preceding clean ups should be done with diligence.

We address their problem on as many levels as we can and as quickly as we can to give them hope and encouragement that the situation can change.

To begin a regimen, the client reads and reviews any materials given them and proceeds to purchase the individual supplements on their regimen. While waiting for their supplements to arrive, they begin a clean up of their living environment. They may start juicing some vegetables for drinks 2 or 3 times a day. They rid their home of any thing they might eat that is not whole, organic, and totally health building by giving those things to a soup kitchen or church pantry (and getting a receipt for all of it!).

Here is the order they begin to follow -

1.   Purchase and assemble all the individual supplements and foods on your particular regimen. Some may be bought locally, and some may have to be bought over the Internet.

2.   Using a craft, sewing, or tackle-type divided box with a multiple of seven compartments, divide out your supplements for one week and for how many times a day you must take your particular supplements. If you take something 3 times a day, the box should contain 21 compartments. If you take something 4 times a day, the box should contain 28 compartments. This will save you a lot of time and can be taken to work or used while traveling.

3.   Do not start your regimen until you assemble all the required items. When starting a full regimen the first day, just take one meal at a time. Get out your supplements and juice or tea (if juice or teas are on your regimen) and take them FIRST. If you still feel hungry, then prepare something that is allowable on your diet sheet for that meal. Many are full the first few days just on the supplements. Do not worry that you are not getting enough nutrition if you do not feel hungry. Some of the supplements you will be taking have enough nutrition to almost make a statue sing!!! If you experience a lack of appetite, your appetite will return within a few days.

4.   SOME, but not ALL, clients experience within the first three to five days SOME of the following things--- nausea, vomiting, leg cramps, arm cramps, stomach cramps, loose stools, headache, parasites in the stool, nasal drainage, a creeping feeling in the muscles, lightheadedness, and sleepiness. DO NOT be alarmed if you experience ANY of these. Your body starts doing a cleansing job as soon as it is given the proper nutrients to do it. If you experience any of these, KEEP ON THE PROGRAM FOR THE NEXT MEAL. These discomforts will soon pass, and you will feel stronger than ever very soon. If you experience anything, it will usually stop by the third day. MOST experience nothing, but feel better from day one. The herbs or supplement are not making you sick... the materials that are being cleansed out by the herbs and supplements are making you sick as they flood your bloodstream and intestines to be eliminated.

5.   If you feel like eating food allowable on your diet sheet after taking your supplements, eat all you need within what is allowable. DO NOT eat anything that is not allowable if you want the full, long-term benefits of the regimen. This is absolutely non-negotiable on the cancer regimen!!!

6.   Be patient with yourself and the regimen. It took you days, weeks, months, or years to get into this condition, and you will be surprised how relatively quickly you can reverse it if you are diligent and consistent.

7.   Make copies of the daily regimen of supplements and diet sheets. You will be handling these many times, and they will get dirty and torn quickly. You could even laminate a copy or two or slip them into a notebook sized clear plastic slipcover.

8.   Start doing the physical clean-up of your home. Remove all household pets and pet related "things", shampoo rugs with a simple soap or remove or replace rugs completely with an hard surface flooring, wash or replace all curtains and drapes, upholstery, and bath and bed linens and pillows, take all chemicals (paints, solvents, etc.) to an outside building, wash the kitchen and bath areas with an anti-bacterial soap such as Palmolive Anti-bacterial dishwashing soap or Dawn Anti-bacterial dishwashing soap or pine oil cleaner (counters, floors, door handles, refrigerator, stove, chairs, dining table, utensils, tub, toilet, sinks, pots, pans, etc.), get air ducts cleaned, and, if possible, buy and use an ionizer (positive and negative)/ozonator).

9.   Buy a juicer and some white Corning ware or other pure glass baking and cooking dishes such as Fire King, Anchor Hocking, Pyrex, or Glasbake.

10.   Have all of your mouth metal removed.

11.   If you can only make your tea or juice once a day, make it in the morning and refrigerate the part to be used later in the day. The tea can be warmed up cup by cup on the stove as needed.

12.   Remember to be very clean in all your food preparation. Wash your hands and utensils frequently and before you start taking out any supplements or food item.

13.   NEVER EAT SPROUTS. Sprout root tips have the gonadotrophic hormone (to grow those root cells rapidly) which is the same hormone that drives cancer cell growth!! NO SPROUTS EVER!

CHAPTER 31

THE ORDER OF RESTORING YOUR HEALTH

There is hardly a health problem that cannot be reversed if all of the organs are there and if proper steps are taken to do the following IN THIS ORDER....

START USING ONLY ORGANIC FOODS, JUICES, TEAS, AND HERBS

USE A VERY CLEAN AND PURE WATER SOURCE

REMOVE HOUSEHOLD PETS FROM THE CONFINED LIVING SPACE

REMOVE TOXIC CHEMICALS FROM THE HOME

SANITIZE THE HOME

RESTORE THE FUNCTION OF THE DIGESTIVE SYSTEM WITH COMPREHENSIVE DIGESTIVE ENZYMES

KILL ALL POSSIBLE PARASITES

KILL THE BACTERIA AND VIRUSES MANUFACTURED AND/OR RESIDING IN AND BEING RELEASED INTO THE BODY BY THE DYING PARASITES WHILE YOU ARE KILLING THE PARASITES

RESTORE THE FUNCTION OF THE BOWEL WITH GENTLE FIBER AND PROBIOTICS

KILL OTHER POSSIBLE PATHOGENS SUCH AS MOLDS AND FUNGI

CLEANSE AND RESTORE THE FUNCTIONING OF THE FILTERING ORGANS (LIVER AND KIDNEY CLEANSES)

CLEANSE CHEMICAL POLLUTANTS IN THE BODY (HERBAL TOXIN CLEANSE)

REPLENISH DEPLETED NUTRIENTS

I have used this order to help clients eliminate some very perplexing problems that even a doctor could not diagnose.

If you follow this order, at some point your symptoms will start dropping away because you are addressing every single possible reason for your symptoms!

Once the client fills out a Client Worksheet, a review is made of their condition and a personalized regimen is made to confront all of their health conditions. Sometimes, it is presented in stages. Sometimes everything is addressed at once.

Some clients want to do all the cleanses at the same time. This is possible and is very intense. AND it brings about results much faster.

Some clients want to do one type of cleanse at a time in succession. This takes longer, but those with small or weak bodies or weak stomachs seem to still do well in the long run approaching things this way.

Some clients can only take the supplements in liquid form. This is also possible until they get stronger.

I have helped some clients who were being fed by a feeding tube. We blended all the supplements in a blender and poured the thinned liquid down the tube.

We used caution to make sure the feeding tube NEVER got clogged by having the nutrients in a thin enough solution. Many get strong enough that the tube can be removed and regular swallowing can resume.

CHAPTER 32

WHAT TO LOOK FOR; WHAT TO EXPECT

As soon as you have assembled all the supplements and utensils needed for the regimen, mark on your calendar Day 1. It is usually a Friday or Saturday (Sabbath). On this day, start taking everything AT LEAST for a Parasite Cleanse and a Viral/Bacterial Cleanse with Comprehensive Digestive Enzymes and multiple probiotics. Take just one meal or supplement time at a time, not thinking about what has to be done all day long. Just take the prepared juices or teas, supplements, and then food, if you have room in your stomach for that meal. Sometimes, and especially at the beginning of the regimen for the first few days, some only take the supplements, juices, and teas. Because your body is adjusting to this new "food" and "medicine" and because your body is starting to clean out, you might be full on these things alone. Some look at this as a partial fast to begin their walk to renewed health.

There are herbal combinations in each of these regimens to deal with "die-off". Die-off is the effects you feel as parasites die and leave viruses, bacteria, molds, and fungi to react in your body. It is the pathogens from the dead parasites flooding your bloodstream and digestive system. If you do not take the herbal combinations to counteract these die-off producers, you may get the worst bacterial infection or viral infection you have ever experienced. Some clients breeze through this possible die-off period. Some experience mild symptoms for 1 to 5 days.

For the first 3 to 5 days, you MAY notice several things. Some people never experience any of these, but you should know about them in case you do experience them WHEN PROCEEDING ON A REGIMEN. These are symptoms of

DIE-OFF. It is the body by the agent of the herbs killing off pathogens in your body.

You may lose your appetite.

You may crave some food very strongly.

You may abruptly lose some long standing craving much to your relief and amazement.

You may have nausea.

You may even vomit your first and second set of supplements or juice as it naturally cleanses your stomach. This is a good thing. Just keep going as scheduled.

You may experience vague cramps in your arms or legs.

You may have more frequent bowel movements, but not diarrhea.

You may experience diarrhea once or twice.

You may have trouble sleeping.

Or you may feel like sleeping all day long!

You may feel more thirsty than usual.

You may have a vague headache.

You may feel a crawling in your tissues as parasites move and die.

As I said before, most people never experience any of these things, but I want you to know, if you have any of these, it is not the herbs causing the problem. It is the foreign chemicals and pathogens you are trying to get rid of finally coming out of your cells, tissues, and organs and going into your blood stream. As pathogens die, the body breaks them down into blood flushable chemicals. The herbs cause the chemicals to come out of hiding and adherence to your cells and into the bloodstream and intestines to be eliminated. Remember, you are ridding your body of things that do not belong there. Of course, you may feel nauseous! These things your body is eliminating are not supposed to be there!

STAY ON THE HERBS AND THE REGIMEN UNTIL THE NAUSEA (or any of the above named possibilities of die-off) stops. This is one of those things that takes FAITH. If you stop the herbs, the die-off symptoms will stop, but the cleansing is not done. You have only stopped the cleansing process. You have to keep up the cleansing process until the nausea or other symptoms stops. Remember, the herbs are not making you nauseous. The dying pathogens and unwanted chemicals are making you nauseous. When all of the offenders are out of your system, the nausea will stop, even if you continue taking the very same herbs!

For me, for example, the nausea (which I hardly ever experienced at any other time) lasted vaguely for about 5 days. It was not a hard nausea, but an "in-the- background-, barely- noticeable" nausea. Over the next 3 weeks once in awhile I felt slight nausea. But there came a point at about 3 weeks when I felt no more nausea, but a feeling of perfect peace inside my body. All of the cravings I had had on and off FOR YEARS WERE GONE and CONTINUE TO BE GONE UNTIL THIS DAY!!

The following is---

CHAPTER 33

MY PERSONAL EXPERIENCE WITH PARASITES

I might not have believed this story unless I had experienced it myself.

My whole life, in every picture of me for as young as I can remember, my stomach stood out. My ballet teacher, from the time I was 5 until I was 16, always was reminding me to "hold in your stomach". I do not remember her ever saying that to all the other students that were in my classes for all those years. Just me! My Dad raised AKC registered dogs that we always let lick our faces, hands, and mouths. We ate all sorts of wild meat my Dad shot like turkey, pheasant, and deer. We ate the fish he caught. We swam in various swimming pools and the Finger Lakes of upstate New York, swallowing the water from time to time.

As a teenager I ate all sorts of Scripturally defined unclean animal flesh such as pork, lobster, raw clams, etc. At times, I let my dog sleep in or on the same bed I slept in. I ate out at various restaurants and at friends' homes without any regard to their cleanliness habits. At age 18, I decided to follow the Creator and a Scriptural diet.

At age 21 and after getting married, I decided to become a lacto-ovo vegetarian. For about 15 years we ate no meat, no white flour, no white sugar. My weight went down to a normal range, my stomach was flatter, but I still always had a little tummy. I always felt hungry. For the next 10 years we ate some meat, some sugar and white flour, but stayed about 80% vegetarian. I started gaining weight. For the next few years I started gaining A LOT of weight, going on the Atkins diet which for me consisted of soybean products, lots of beef, turkey, tuna, fish, and lots of eggs and cheeses. I sometimes felt dizzy and light headed although I was getting adequate calories and protein.

I still gained weight after losing about 30 pounds on this diet. I started having digestive problems. I felt something moving up and down my large intestine. I broke out with large brown blotches all over my face. I started having pain in my knees, shoulders, ankles, toes, and fingers. I started having frequent headaches, something I never experienced before. I heard frequent sounds in my digestive tract that I had never heard before. I felt something crawling up my throat, it seemed, from my stomach to my lungs. I had very bad breath and very dry stools. I had rapid heart beat. Sometimes after eating, in a few minutes, I had a terrible pain at the top of my stomach that felt like a strong pinching feeling. I also felt this pinching feeling from time to time just above my appendix. At night I would wake up with night sweating and rapid heartbeat and noises in my throat. I felt something crawling at times from my anus to my vagina. I had lumps in the muscles in my arms and above my knees and just below my knees that were very hard.

I had put my clients on parasite cleanses for YEARS, but had never really done a thorough one on myself. I decided one day to treat myself for cancer, parasites, and Chagas disease all at one time. In spite of my never having been in a tropical country, I was bitten by a strange bug on my eyelid and after the bite, I developed every symptom of Chagas disease while living in North Carolina. Up to this point I had regular bowel movements that were well formed, effortless, and odorless. But they slowly turned very dry and hard. AND there was a line all along the side of each stool that puzzled me after I noticed it accidentally one day.

I started on the regimen.....

Within a week, I passed in my stool the following.... 3 liver flukes about 2 inches long, another kind of fluke about 1½ inches long, a one foot LONG red worm and accompanying gunk attached to it that looked like liver material, 2 one foot long hookworms, small rice grain size worms, 3 cancer fungal "fuzzies" (these look like black koosh balls about the size of a ping pong ball and are usually present when colon cancer is growing), dozens of black stringy worms each about 3 inches long, about 20 light colored parasites that looked like small stacked French fries and balls of something that looked like nearly clear small pearl onions. I passed a lot of the liver looking material.

The smell was sickening. I never smelled these smells before. My breath was terrible tasting. And I kept smelling dead flesh from time to time in my nose and throat. I coughed up nasty stuff from my lungs and stomach and spit it out. Anytime I smelled any type of meat I got terribly nauseous. But I kept on the regimen.

The first indication of my passing a parasite was when I went to use the toilet about the third day and after wiping myself there was about a 6 inch grayish, yellowish, bluish thing that looked like a flattened piece of pasta still hanging out of me. I pulled on it with toilet paper and it was attached, with pain, at the spot just above my appendix that frequently pinched. I now figured out that the pinching was a worm grabbing on tighter or at a close by position from time to time. Now I knew I must also have a hookworm at the top of my stomach from the similarity of the pinching pains. Then I passed all the things mentioned above in about 2 or 3 days. There were several drops of blood in my stool, probably from where the worms detached.

After about 3 weeks I did not see any unusual things in my stool anymore. I had lost all desire for meat. I had lost all desire for dairy products. I had lost all desire for anything sweet. And my stomach was almost perfectly flat. As a matter of fact, I hardly felt like eating anything, being perfectly at peace with my body and having no cravings that I had had for months. I lost 15 pounds in about a month. I felt so peaceful. I had no nagging appetite that I had had for YEARS! Let me repeat... I had no nagging appetite and had lost all my vague cravings for any and all foods in sight I had had for YEARS. I went several days without even THINKING about eating and yet was totally at peace with my body. I still, for about a month, would smell rotting flesh in my nose and throat. I think that some of the parasites in my sinuses, upper stomach, and lungs were dead and slowly decaying.

All of the diabetic type symptoms I had experienced before were gone and I had steady even energy all day long without the ups and downs and hunger spurts from before. All of the symptoms of Chagas disease that I had experienced were gone, also. The irregular, and sometimes fast, heartbeat, the sour stomach, the typical swollen eyelid, the constant choking feeling, and the night sweats were all gone. Almost all of the brown patches all over my face were gone!! The dark circles and yellowish skin tone were gone. The pain and aches in ALL of my joints was gone. For several years I had a feeling of claustrophobia from time to time. It was now gone.

Here is what I took...

Parasite killing herb capsules - 10 caps in the morning
Colonix - 1 scoop plus 1 T. Equate powder later in the day
Neem capsules - 2 caps 3 times a day-Penn Herb or www.thebesorahseed.com
Turmeric capsules –2 caps 3 times a day (homemade from grocery store turmeric)
Essiac capsules – 4 caps 2 times a day (homemade from 4 Herb Formula from Herbal Healer Academy)
Garlic capsules – 2 tabs 3 times a day (KYOLIC #100, #101, or #102)

MSM – 1500 mgs. (Wal-Mart)

Carrot juice, sometimes with parsley juice – 2 glasses a day

Buried Treasure ACF – 1 T. 3 times a day

500 PPM Colloidal Silver - 1 T. 3 times a day from Herbal Healer Academy

Selenium – 200 mcgs. tablet

RM 10 – by Garden of Life – 4 a day

Co-enzyme Q-10 -3 grams or 3,000 mgs a day for 3 days

I ate a vegan diet. I ate lots of cucumbers, parsley, pumpkin seeds, and cilantro. I drank carrot and parsley juice, and pomegranate juice as all these things also kill parasites.

YOU CAN HAVE DRAMATIC RESULTS LIKE THIS IF YOU FOLLOW THE PRINCIPLES OUTLINED IN THIS BOOK.

NEAR THE END OF THE BOOK ARE VERY SPECIFIC REGIMENS YOU CAN FOLLOW TO GET EXCELLENT RESULTS-- THE SAME RESULTS AS HUNDREDS OF MY CLIENTS HAVE EXPERIENCED!

CHAPTER 34

DEAL WITH YOUR CRAVINGS AND ADDICTIONS

Cravings are a Creator given sign to us, just as thirst is a sign to you that you need more water and tiredness or sleepiness is a sign that you need to go to sleep and rest.

If you have cravings, you have to be a detective and define your cravings.

Do you crave dairy foods?

Do you crave sugar?

Do you crave greasy foods?

Do you crave carrots?

Do you crave broccoli?

Do you crave meat, meat, meat?

Do you crave something you just cannot define, but you just keep eating hoping the craving will go away?

A craving indicates your body needs more of something it is not receiving on the cellular level, just as thirst indicates your cells are not receiving enough water.

Cravings can be a genuine knowing for something YOU need for YOUR BODY, but they also can be a genuine craving a PARASITE NEEDS to keep living in your body. Let me explain.

A human needs about 60 grams of complete protein a day to function normally, even if exercising heavily. If you are well and not hosting any parasites, this amount will completely satisfy you. And some days, it will even seem like too much protein. But if you have meat (or protein)-craving parasites, they will take nearly all the protein you put into your digestive tract that they need to survive before it any of the protein gets a chance to get to YOUR cells! They ALWAYS get the best of what you eat and you are left with the LEFTOVERS OR NONE AT ALL! Therefore, you may have eaten protein in the form of meat, but very little of it or none may have actually gotten to your cells; therefore you crave meat AND PROTEIN to fill YOUR needs. The more you eat, the more they thrive and multiply if there, and the less actually gets to your cells making you crave and crave and consume and consume even more!

Now try going on a diet under these conditions! It is an absolutely miserable and futile thing to do! You feel weaker by the day because the less you consume, the more percentage-wise the parasites are getting of your food so your energy level plummets, discouraging you from day one. This is one of the main reasons people quit reducing diets!

There are dairy foods craving parasites. There are sugar craving parasites. There are parasites that sap you of every micronutrient that you cannot define like selenium, boron, chromium, etc. Because our food supply is so depleted in these micronutrients TO BEGIN WITH, we eat foods that we hope will stop these cravings, but even after eating what we absolutely know is enough calories, we are still craving SOMETHING. This is what leads to the vast overeating some people feel is beyond their control. And uncontrolled weight gain.

One particular client told me she had been held captive by sugar cravings for as long as she could remember. She was really being held captive by her sugar craving parasites that had been living inside of her most likely since birth or early childhood. She said the cravings she had were so strong and so totally dominated her every day and her thinking for as far back as she could remember that she wondered if she was demonically possessed. After a thorough herbal parasite cleanse, she said she was free for the first time (in 60 years!) in her life of this craving.

I have had the same experience and so have many of my clients. A good parasite cleanse frees you from the parasites and these cravings and finally your body gets the nutrients it needs with no competition from the parasites.

There are cravings your body can have without parasites being the cause. If you crave any particular food, you probably have a deficiency of a nutrient in that food. This is why pregnant ladies have weird cravings. The baby is taking the best of what the mother is consuming. The mother's body only gets the leftovers. When she eats the foods she craves, it replenishes what she needs for herself.

When I was pregnant with our twins, every night between 3 AM and 5 AM, I would wake up craving the exact same thing. Canned salmon with mayonnaise, red pepper (cayenne), and yellow nutritional yeast all mixed together. I can barely stand to even look at that combination now, but I craved it, and it satisfied me every time I ate it. As soon as the twins were born, I stopped craving it.

One winter, I craved Brazil nuts. I used to hate Brazil nuts. I always avoided Brazil nuts in a mixed nut bowl. But that winter, I could not get enough of Brazil nuts. As soon as spring came, I stopped having the cravings.

I remember in my basic nutrition class at Cornell the professor telling of a study done at a college with a department of nutrition. They allowed toddlers to crawl for one month for 3 meals a day down a cafeteria serving line. In this line was food from every food group. They let the toddlers eat whatever they wanted. Each child was watched carefully, and all they ate was recorded.

Some ate about the same thing each day. Some gorged on some foods at different times and seemed to crave certain things completely passing by some other foods. One toddler stuffed a lot of salt in his mouth just one day. But at the end of the month, when the records were checked, each toddler had eaten approximately the same amount of each food in each group. In other words, their cravings, if satisfied, eventually equaled out to a healthy, balanced diet.

One reminder about cravings!!! If you crave unhealthy foods or unclean meats, it is not you craving these, it is your microbes (and most likely those microbes are parasites), craving these things. A healthy body, free from pathogens, craves very good and Scripturally clean foods. After all, it was designed by the Creator to crave only these foods when in need. If you are craving a natural food like broccoli, oranges, figs, greens, or the like, by all means, fill that craving! If you are craving greasy French fries, an over load of meat, soda pop, candy, sugary baked goods, etc., do not fill that craving. Instead, take a parasite cleanse!

Just as thirst tells you how much water you need, true cravings are a signal you are missing something in your diet. If you can not define those cravings, you may be missing some trace minerals in your diet. A good mixed green supplement (Organifi Green, Green Vibrance, Perfect Food, Marine Greens, 6 Seaweed Formula Capsules from Naturespirit Herbs, etc.) with several sea greens in the formula will supply all the trace minerals you may be craving. Start taking these AFTER you take a parasite cleanse.

Many clients have told me their cravings and addictions faded after going on this program. It addresses all the possible robbers of nutrition and adds in nutrients where there has been a deficiency.

ADDICTIONS

There are some very specific nutrients that need to be added in specific addictions. Smoking uses up much B complex vitamins and Vitamin C. Alcohol uses much B complex vitamins, calcium, and magnesium. Recreational drugs use up much calcium, magnesium, protein, B complex vitamins, and Vitamin C. Some addicts stop eating all together. These cases need all of the above plus a very comprehensive organic multimineral and multivitamin to fill in all the deficiencies.

We had a friend who owned a health food store in Brooklyn, New York. He told me the people applying for city jobs always had to take drug tests before actually going to work for the city. He said he had people come in to the store all the time asking for something to clear the drugs out of their bloodstreams before the test. He gave them golden seal root capsules. This blood cleanser can pull all traces of the drugs out.

I suggest a combination similar to this to pull some of the harmful effects out of the blood stream when a person had decided not to use drugs any more. It helps the withdrawal and speeds recovery to use these herbs. If a person is going "cold turkey", using valerian eases the cramping and jitters of the withdrawal. Golden seal leaves or root, burdock root, chickweed, dandelion, hyssop, red clover, sanicle or blue sanicle, sorrel, yellow dock, borage, echinacea, organic dark blue grape juice, and others all pull foreign chemicals out of the blood and tissues. These are effective for removing recreational drugs and their effects, conventional medical drugs, chemotherapy, and some kinds of poisoning. Activated charcoals, however, is the safest and quickest to act of any poison control.

Each client has to be evaluated individually for their specific addiction and deficiencies.

CHAPTER 35

OBESITY

What if we find out it really IS hormones? What if we find out it is caused by all the chemicals put on our foods? What if we find out it is the pesticides we consume? What if we find out it is the half foods we are eating? What if we find out it is that we are not moving for our life? What if it is really caused by parasites?

What if we find out the sweetest, most feminine ladies have a chemical imbalance of estrogen that causes them to store fat at higher rates than others? What if we find out cow's milk causes humans to grow to cow like proportions? What if it is confirmed that certain mutated bacteria or viruses make fat cells grow unchecked?

How is it that a person can lose weight through reduced calorie intake and hours of exercise and then very quickly regain all they lost and more? How is it that so many are so resistant to losing large amounts of weight? How is it that we eat so many more calories than we need and still have little or no energy to use for daily activities?

These are all questions we need to ask.

Here are a few thoughts.

Many pesticides have an estrogen-like chemical in them. Too much estrogen or an imbalance of the three estrogens normally produced by the HUMAN body(MALE AND FEMALE!) causes the body to store more fat instead of burn calories for energy. This estrogen imbalance can affect men and women.

Dr. Amen has a tape series and book named CHANGE YOUR BRAIN, CHANGE YOUR BODY that goes into the many, many reasons beyond calories in, calories out that causes this generation to be overweight. There are many factors that many people do not know anything about. His book is definitely worth reading, taking notes on, and implementing his evidence based suggestions.

In a former chapter I mentioned the role of parasites in keeping weight high. Parasites can so distort your appetite that to try to go on a diet is failure from day one. Get rid of parasites first, then start being more moderate in your eating.

Parasites in the thyroid and pancreas can also affect weight gain and inability to lose weight.

Things that have really helped people lose weight...Parasite and viral cleanses, liver flushes, colon refurbishing, more organic protein, fresh spinach, apple cider vinegar, addition of chromium to the diet, drinking more pure water, drink one quart of water upon arising, walk one or two hours a day outside in the fresh air and sunshine, carrot juice, greens juices, water aerobics, dancing, bounce on a mini trampoline for a minute or two several times a day, zumba, stretching, sleeping at least 7 hours in total darkness, African mango, garcinia cambogia, citrus essential oils, omega oils, citrifolia, l-carnitine, kelp, etc.

CHAPTER 36

PREGNANT MOTHERS

THE GREATEST GIFT YOU CAN GIVE YOUR UNBORN CHILD

JUST EAT REAL FOOD DURING PREGNANCY AND LOTS OF VARIETIES OF FOODS.

There are many steps in your baby's development in your womb. If you skip a step or do not have the right nutrients right there available every day to be used in this process of building your baby's body, you can never recover or retrace your steps to do it right the second time. It is so important expectant mothers understand this. You must have adequate nutrients available at all times during pregnancy. A diet with a lot of variety and a good organic pre-natal supplement taken every day will help supply all the nutrients your baby needs for optimum genetic growth. A good diet allows for the baby's body to grow to the fullest of its genetic potential at every stage of development.

One day I had a yard sale when my 8 children were little. A girl came to the sale. We talked a little and she said, "Would you like to see my new baby?" Of course I did and we walked over to her car. In the car seat was a perfectly beautiful little girl with no fingers or toes! I was shocked! I told the Mom how beautiful she was. I asked her, "What types of things do you like to eat?" She told me, "Hamburgers and grapes and sometimes mashed potatoes." I asked her, "Is that all? What else do you like to eat?" She said, "That is all I really like." I asked her, "Did you take a prenatal vitamin during pregnancy?" She said, "No." I told her, "The next time you get pregnant, please eat more different types of foods and lots of salads and fruits, vegetables, nuts, milk of some kind, and whole grain bread."

I am so concerned about today's young mothers and their babies–to-be. They have grown up on empty junk foods. They have eaten foods loaded with non-food chemicals. Their parents have had them take multiple antibiotics and multiple vaccinations as they grew up. They have used over the counter drugs like Pez candies. They have used recreational drugs like birthday cake. They eat the same greasy and sugary foods day in and day out. What does this generation have in storage for the next generation, nutritionally?

When my oldest daughter married and became pregnant, she lost her first pregnancy of twins in the early stages. At that time, she started telling me that nearly every young married girl she knew lost their first pregnancy spontaneously. She listed off many, many girls we both knew and I was perplexed. I wondered if this was the body's way of cleansing all the toxic pollutant chemicals from the uterus. Most of those girls had perfectly successful second pregnancies.

We are having more defects per thousand newborns than ever recorded in the USA. We have more defects per thousand than countries where a simple, monotonous, more whole foods diet is the mainstay!!

The reason for these defects is not genetic. Most people who have a miscarriage can eventually have at least one or more successful pregnancies. Mothers who drastically improve and diversify their diets produce perfectly healthy and whole children. It is the chemicals in the water, food, drinks, the pollution in the air, the multiple over the counter drugs, the recreational drugs,the vaccinations, and the multiplier effect of all these chemicals working together to logjam, interrupt, or stop regularly occurring chemical processes that have to proceed unhindered if the thousands of steps to produce a healthy baby is to be the final result.

This is because of all the chemicals in and on the foods and lack of nutrients in the Mother's nutritional storage bank. One of the best books on this subject, showing conclusively that how you eat several months prior to and during pregnancy determines the beauty (symmetrical formation of bones and teeth), intelligence (proper formation of brain and nerve tissue), and demeanor (formation of nervous, spine, and brain tissues and synapses) are absolutely determined by what you eat and the nutrients available at each stage of fetal development, is LET'S HAVE HEALTHY CHILDREN by Adelle Davis. Every woman wanting to get pregnant should read this book at least 6 months before she plans on getting pregnant. Following the evidence based advice of this book will save the child, the parents, the school system, the church, the legal system, the insurance companies, the penal system, the grandparents tremendous misery, expense, and heartache if followed. What you put in your mouth (or do not put in), is what you are going to get in a newborn baby's body.

In January 2011, a report came out that "pretty" people have higher intelligence. That makes perfect sense to me. "Pretty" people have more symmetric features. That is what makes them "pretty"! If you have more symmetric features, it means you had very adequate pre-natal nutrition to be able to form equally as well on both sides of your body. It also means there was very adequate nutrition for all of your brain tissue to form, hence pretty people have higher intelligence. Adelle Davis found this to be true, also.

I had a very dear friend who was a pediatric nurse who understood pre-natal nutrition very well. Her son married a beautiful but immature girl who became pregnant. All the girl would eat during pregnancy was tin canned sugar cookies. She felt terrible during the pregnancy. Her tender beauty failed. She delivered a live child with MULTIPLE defects. Thousands upon thousands of dollars of corrective surgeries were needed for that child. The mother became pregnant again and followed nearly the same diet. The second little girl had the same and worse defects!

Once you get pregnant, it is not about you anymore. It is about your child. Your life, your body is the vessel to grow another totally independently functioning human being. You are totally responsible as much as you can control to make sure your diet is adequate enough to cover all of your child's growing needs.

HOW YOU EAT DURING PREGNANCY DETERMINES A LOT OF WHAT THAT CHILD'S LIFE IS GOING TO BE ALL ABOUT IN THE FUTURE. How you eat determines how clearly he is going to be able to think AND PROCESS WHAT IS GOING ON IN THIS WORLD. How you eat is going to determine how good looking that child is. How you eat is going to determine how calm or antsy his demeanor is, SETTING A PATTERN FOR HIM IN EVERY GROUP HE ENCOUNTERS UNTIL HE DIES.

MANY YOUNG GIRLS EAT ONLY A FEW OF THE SAME FOODS DAY IN AND DAY OUT. They eat the same thing every day. This is the reason their babies are not formed right. You have to switch up and get many types of foods to get all the nutrients you and your baby need during pregnancy. You need...

1. A very good calcium/magnesium/Vitamin D/boron supplement for your baby's bones, teeth, and jaws to form properly.

2. Plus a good greens or seaweed supplement for trace minerals

3. Plus a comprehensive natural and organic pre-natal supplement in order to give enough nutrition to your body for all your child needs in this polluted environment. And take twice as much if you are carrying twins!

4. Garden of Life Raw Probiotics, Coromega orange, hazelnuts, sesame seeds, and carrot juice.

Zinc is just one thing necessary for the child's reproductive system to form normally. Children of pregnant mothers who took zinc during pregnancies have larger reproductive organs and fewer reproductive problems later on in life.

Forget greasy foods, but do eat some avocado, nuts, seeds, or natural oils every day. I ate a lot of sesame seed butter (tahini) in every (7 successful) pregnancy as it has nutrients to form the brain well.

MY HUSBAND AND I WANTED A LARGE FAMILY. I BIRTHED 8 CHILDREN IN 12 YEARS. My last successful pregnancy was twin girls. In between all of those pregnancies, I was breast feeding. I understood at that time that there was like a faucet turned on full blast of nutrients exiting my body by being either pregnant or nursing for 12 years straight. I took handfuls of supplements of all kinds to make sure I had enough to keep going personally as well as have an abundance of nutrients to give to my unborn children. I ate as many varieties of foods as we had available. All of my 8 children had high IQ's and nearly perfect bone formation, large healthy teeth, and a calm demeanor. If you want a perfectly formed, beautiful, alert, calm, smart child, you have to eat a huge variety of foods. Look at pregnancy as an adventure to try all sorts of new, but organic, raw and natural foods.

ORGANIC IS ALWAYS BEST!

SAMPLE ALL THE FRUITS

SAMPLE ALL THE VEGETABLES

SAMPLE ALL THE GLUTEN FREE GRAINS

SAMPLE ALL THE SEEDS

SAMPLE ALL THE GREENS

SAMPLE ALL THE ROOT VEGETABLES

EAT SEA GREENS IN SOME FORM

TAKE A GOOD ORGANIC PRE-NATAL SUPPLEMENT

TAKE A CALCIUM/MAGNESIUM/VITAMIN D/BORON SUPPLEMENT

NOTE! DO NOT USE GMO BASED TAMPONS OR DIAPERS! THESE FIBERS CAUSE MANY PROBLEMS INSIDE AND OUTSIDE THE BODY. USE ORGANIC TAMPONS AND ORGANIC DIAPERS- WHETHER CLOTH OR PAPER! AMAZON .COM AND WWW.VITACOST.COM EACH HAVE BOTH!

CHAPTER 37

WIVES AND MOTHERS

THE GREATEST SERVICE A MOTHER CAN GIVE HER HUSBAND AND
GROWING CHILDREN

What you as a mother feed your family TODAY determines their BEHAVIOUR
and HEALTH TOMORROW and in some cases, in the NEXT FEW MINUTES, the
NEXT FEW HOURS, the NEXT FEW DAYS, the NEXT FEW WEEKS, and the
NEXT FEW MONTHS when confronted with passing community pathogens (flu,
viruses, bacterial infections), their long term health in the form of whether they
will develop degenerative disease, and the actual number of days they will live.
Now is there any reason why ANY MOTHER should feel INSIGNIFICANT
anymore?

The reason for this is that what you eat and how you treat your body has
CUMULATIVE EFFECTS. It is not just what you do right now that gives you
good health. You reap what you have sown in the past. Only with starting
TODAY can you build a history to rely on for your long term health IN THE
FUTURE if you have failed in the past. Some failures we are ignorant of. Other
failures we are TOTALLY responsible for because we just purposely made bad
choices! Even still, however, the Scripture says, "the curse causeless shall not
come" (Proverbs 26:2)

Many times we wonder why some seemingly good people have bad things
happen to them—especially in the health area. Most likely they are reaping
what they have sown in their past health life. Just because we do not see the
cliff behind the bushes, does not prevent us from falling over the cliff when we
crash through the bushes. The cliff was there whether we saw it or not.

162

We have all heard it told and most likely said it ourselves, "All the answers to life are in the Scriptures." and yet we are not alert enough to realize, ALL the answers to LIFE ARE in the Scriptures! The Creator told us from the beginning how to eat. Are we doing what He said to do?

Your family's health TODAY AND TOMORROW is determined by what you fed them yesterday or today. Are there enough nutrients in today's meals to help them grow in the stage of growth they are in today, confront stress successfully with patience, allow their nerves and brain to presently function properly, as well as put a little nutrition in storage for the future stresses? All of this and more are determined by what you fed them yesterday and today.

What you fed them today starts a pattern of eating that will end up as a life long pattern of eating if it does not change by your doing or theirs. We simply eat as our family always does and as always has without thinking.

What they are fed today determines your doctor and health and possibly your hospital bills in the future. If you do not think that is true, follow several people who have been hospitalized with heart attacks in their 40's and ask them what they ate as children.

If they are not fed adequate nutrition on a daily basis, giving enough for the day's stresses and growth plus some for storage, they will succumb to every illness that passes in the community and in the air. When a sickness passes through a population, you will notice not everyone gets it, even some of those who work with the VERY sickest. Those who have some storage of nutrients FOR THEIR IMMUNE SYSTEM to help mount a successful battle against a sickness IN THE FUTURE are the ones who do not fall ill. This is how poor diet fails your family in short-term illnesses.

Continual bad diet, over months and years, sets the stage for degenerative diseases. Degenerative diseases are those that can be easily prevented or even reversed by adequate nutrition. It is obvious that if nutrition were adequate every day with even some left over for storage, degenerative disease would be non-existent! This is how premature aging, continual short term illnesses, de-mineralization of the bones and teeth, loss of function in the organs and tissues and other conditions are prevented.

Bad food, Bad Food, BAD FOOD day in and day out stresses the body so much that it shortens the days on earth. How many of us have seen people who smoke 4 packs of cigarettes a day and live only to 35 or 45? How many of us have known people who eat pork and pies, and greasy foods and candy all day long and die in their 40's? How many of us have sadly seen beautiful young people become all wrinkles and sallow by the ravages of drugs and alcohol and die premature deaths?

I have seen women who were gorgeous in the teens and 20's look like they are in their 50's by the time they are 35! They smoked, drank diet soda continuously, ate greasy foods and white bread and hardly ANY fresh fruits and vegetables. They suffered aging effects like a woman in her 70's from the self deprivation of nutrients. It all has to do with their diet and ability to handle daily stress with their diet. You can take tremendous stress if your diet is adequate to cover the stress.

The body is programmed by the Creator at this point in history to live between 70 and 120 years if organically fed. There are many cultures where the majority of the populations live well past 100 EVEN IN THIS POLLUTED WORLD! So we do have that possibility of living longer than we think and see, in very good shape if we put forth the effort to make it so.

Do not be deceived by all that is offered as food. Only organic, whole fresh (or dried or frozen or pickled) foods are REAL food. Only those that are absolutely free of any applied non-food chemicals are the real things that can repair, refresh, AND PROLONG THE LIFE OF your body.

So, this very serious business of keeping in your home only that which is health building and preparing for your family only those things which are sufficient for today with some left for health "insurance" for the future is a VERY BIG MINISTRY with far reaching consequences. Shifting this responsibility to restaurants, fast food places, commercial bakeries, and candy manufacturers is a "cop out". Just as it is the parent's responsibility to feed their children spiritually those things that will benefit them spiritually, it is the parent's responsibility to feed their children physically only those things that will benefit their bodies physically. Just as it is the parent's responsibility to keep out of their home any thing that would harm their child or family, so is it their responsibility to keep out any thing masquerading as "food".

How many young mothers say it drives them crazy that their children are always so loud and uncontrollable as they feed them sugar, artificial flavors, and artificial colors? The answer to their questions is in their hands and under their control!

Only REAL FOOD is REAL FOOD for your growing child's body!

You do not have to make everything from "scratch". There are some companies that are trustworthy enough to only put wholesome ingredients in their prepared foods. Walnut Acres, Purely Decadent, Full Circle, Arrowhead Mills, Rudi's Organics, Health Valley Organics, Muir Glen and many more have long established reputations of continually having a conscience of putting only good whole, organic ingredients in their foods. Some grocery chains now have their own brands of organic foods. Read the labels of EVERYTHING you purchase. BY NOT BUYING A PRODUCT YOU SEND A MESSAGE TO THE MANUFACTURER THAT YOU ARE LOOKING FOR SOMETHING BETTER THAN THEIR PRODUCT or the same product at a cheaper price! Do not waste your hard earned money on something that is going to eventually kill you or your family!

In the small community where I live, I have to shop between 3 different stores to get all I need to make up meals for my family that contain only whole, wholesome, organic ingredients. It takes about a half a workday a week to go to all these stores and sort through what they have available TODAY for me to stock my kitchen for the next few days. It takes patience and perseverance to do this. But I have always tried to get the best so my family could have the best health possible. There have been times when very few organic groceries were even for sale in this community (as I am sure is the case in many communities).

Grow your own food. Buy at local farmer's markets only the organic offerings. Organize a community garden where the entire work load is not just on one person or one family. START an organic coop where you and several friends buy organic foods in bulk and split shipments among yourselves. Order in bulk from places like www.nuts.com or www.vitacost.com. Tell your friends whose children play with your children that you all NEED to feed the children better and ask them to help you and you help them to provide only health building foods and snacks in your neighborhood. Speak up in friendly sincere tones! It can be done!

KICK SUGAR OUT OF YOUR DIET

If you really knew what sugar did to your body and your family member's bodies, you would never touch it again! It is a poison of sorts; it is addictive as any drug. It is totally devoid of nutrients that help your body. Get rid of sugar completely. Use date sugar or honey or maple syrup in great moderation. Use stevia sparingly. Avoid artificial sweeteners like a plague. Get your children hooked on fruits and vegetables for snacks. Use seeds and nuts more frequently. Give your children water to drink 9 times out of 10 even before organic fruit juices. The books SWEET AND DANGEROUS by John Yudkin or SUICIDE BY SUGAR by Nancy Appleton tell the astonishing facts about the deadly effects of eating sugar regularly.

An interesting fact - I read an article recently where it told that wealthy people in the 1700's and 1800's had "sugar" parties where all they ate was sugar and they experienced highs (or hyperactivity) nearly the same as the cocaine parties people have now! That is what it did to bodies that were not used to it on a daily basis!

WIPE OUT GREASE

Stay away from fried foods. This generation eats way too much grease in French fries and chicken nuggets. This greasy food is so hard on your child's delicate digestive system. I am so alarmed about just this one horrible eating habit. It is hard enough on ADULT digestive systems. How much more harmful is it to children's DEVELOPING digestive systems????

Greasy foods plus sugary ANYTHING (soda, candy, cakes, pies, cookies, ice cream, etc.) plus white bread form a gluey substance that accumulates in your intestines. It hardens over time and slowly kills the function of your intestines. It ends up like cement in your intestines and slowly fills the intestine from the outside in until there is only a small hole for food to pass down the length of the digestive tract. The actual food gets farther and farther away from the intestinal wall where its NUTRIENTS ARE SUPPOSED TO BE ABSORBED but can not as it can not touch the walls of the intestine anymore. Now the whole body starts starving because it can not get the nutrients into the circulatory system to feed the whole body!

Kick out these robbers of your and your children's health. Feed the whole family REAL FOOD!

WHITE BREAD IS FOR THE BIRDS! (POOR BIRDS!)

Stop buying AND EATING white bread. It is an absolute killer. Take a piece of white bread and squish it down to a cube or roll it into a ball. This is what it does in your intestines. It forms gluey balls and blocks the intestines so they can not work properly. It is a colon CLOGGER. Whole grain breads, however, are colon CLEANERS. Start with whole grains as soon as your child can eat solid foods. View white sugar, white flour, and white rice as killers because, in the long run, THEY ARE!!!

Oh, yes, by the way!!! I have actually seen birds at feeding ponds refuse to eat white bread!

"You better think"   - Aretha Franklin

I hate sickness. I hate being sick, and I hate to see my loved ones sick. Besides feeling so sorry for them for their pain and misery, it is such a time waster. And sometimes so unnecessary. And sometimes the cause is so selfish. Someone who eats poorly just for taste or someone who refuses to wash their hands when appropriate or someone who is just too lazy to cover their mouth when they sneeze or cough can all cause hardship on others and give opportunity for disease to spread further, doing even more damage, wasting time, and slowing productivity and progress.

Children and adults need to be taught these things of the way to better health and to be shown a good example without complaining in this area. The parents decide what comes into the house for the family in the way of food and training. Make sure everything you bring in the home is good for everyone in the home, physically and spiritually. It is so RESTFUL AND REWARDING to have children who are calm, healthy, and so welcoming to eating real, whole foods when they have been raised on them.

The parents set the pace. The parents set the example. The parents buy the food. Get yourself under control by taking care of your health so you can be an example for your children. If you need to take some of these cleanses TO GET YOUR OWN DIET UNDER CONTROL before you address your whole family's food supply, do it so you can BE THE EXAMPLE.

We all have learned many things from our parents, grandparents, the world, and our taking examples and lessons from our observations of this world. Some were good and some were bad. It is now our responsibility to correct ourselves according to REAL truth for ourselves and for the future generations. It is time you now take as an example the Scriptures and adjust and fine tune your life according to its teachings.

I have often thought how if a woman cooks and feeds her husband and children pies, cakes, "shortening", and grease for years she is actually participating in "shortening" their lives. Choices made today affect happenings in the future! Choose wisely and in love for the best for your loved ones.

CHAPTER 38

HOW TO STOP ALCOHOL CRAVING

Dr. Hulda Clark has discovered in her research the true cause and cure for alcohol craving. It is NOT a social disease. It is NOT a character defect. It is NOT an acquired habit. It is a combination of a chemical pollutant and mold that occupy the pleasure producing part of the brain that causes the craving for alcohol. This chemical and mold can be passed to a child while in the mother's womb. Using an all natural supplement regimen, the desire for alcohol and all its deadly side effects can be permanently eliminated in a few days. This has helped many, many people become permanently alcohol free using these discoveries.

Dr. Clark found the element beryllium usually is eliminated by the liver, but when the liver is disabled or over taxed, the chemical circulates freely in the bloodstream. She found that the chemical beryllium (found in coal products, coal oil, gasoline, kerosene, hurricane lamp oil, hurricane lamps, antique lamps, paint solvents, automotive products, paint cleaners, solvent cleaners, cigarette lighters, dry cleaning fumes, etc.) circulates in the bloodstream and lands at the addiction center of the brain (this center produces the pleasure sensing chemicals). This chemical is very reactive with alcohol. The two together in the brain cause certain neurotransmitters in the brain to be released that should not be released and restrict the release of neurotransmitters that should be released. This brings on the high or the depression of the alcoholic condition.

She also found that a mold common in food and alcoholic beverages (ergot mold) works with alcohol at the addiction center to make each other more toxic and reactive.

The pleasure producing part of the brain is usually carefully controlled by other chemicals so that not too much pleasure or happiness can be experienced. The site where the offending beryllium can land is normally the site for glutamate. When glutamate can not land there, the joy and happiness center cannot function, producing low level chronic depression and the craving for a time out of the depression, which translates into a craving for alcohol. The more beryllium present, the worse the depression. Supplementing the diet with glutamine (which the body turns into glutamate) helps boot out the beryllium. (It has been found that at least 3 grams of glutamine should be taken daily by those with depression and alcohol craving.)

When alcohol is put on the skin (tinctures, lotions, aftershaves, colognes, gasoline, petroleum solvents, etc.), inhaled, or put in the mouth (mouthwashes, OTC medicines, alcoholic beverages, etc.) or produced in the intestines by fermentation (as by Candida yeast), a substance named salsol is formed. Salsol reacts very quickly with beryllium. At the pleasure producing site, the two together produce large quantities of pleasure producing chemicals. This is the alcoholic "high". You can feel this alcoholic "high" without ever drinking an alcoholic beverage if you have a Candida yeast infection in your intestines!!

As the beryllium is removed by natural means (by glutamine and by thioctic acid [otherwise known as alpha lipoic acid]), the salsol also disappears.

In order to eliminate the depressions in between alcoholic highs, to regulate the normal sense of well being and happiness without alcoholic consumption, and to eliminate the craving for alcohol, two things have to be avoided and eliminated from the body- beryllium and ergot mold. 10 grams (or 10,000 mgs. of Vitamin C- ester, buffered) in 3 divided doses daily will destroy the ergot. Taking at least 3 grams of glutamine daily and 600 mgs. alpha lipoic acid daily will remove the beryllium and salsol. An high B-complex tablet (B-75 or B-100) and 500 mgs. niacin amide taken 3 times a day will help the neurotransmitters to recover quickly. A GOOD, COMPREHENSIVE MULTI-VITAMIN AND MULTI-MINERAL SUPPLEMENT IS ALSO RECOMMENDED TO HELP FILL IN ALL NUTRITIONAL DEFICIENCIES CAUSED BY ALCOHOL CONSUMPTION. Green Vibrance, Natural Vitality Organic Life liquid, or Buried Treasure VM-100 are three formulas.

If you have no ergot or beryllium, and yet force yourself to consume alcohol, you will still have impaired brain and neurological responses from the alcohol alone. But the constant craving will not be there, if the ergot and beryllium are eliminated. This is another and different problem that should be dealt with.

Some people drink alcohol just for the lightheaded, reality subduing feeling, not to fulfill a craving. But if alcohol is consumed regularly even for THIS reason, there is still much brain and liver damage, as well as multiple nutritional deficiencies created. IF YOU HAVE PROBLEMS YOU NEED TO DEAL WITH, GET HELP FROM A SCRIPTURAL COUNSELOR. If there is some reality you are trying to escape, get away from the source, if possible. If you are constantly receiving negative messages from someone close to you, remove yourself from their presence. If you are tired, get more rest. If you tire too quickly on your job you must work, find out the foods and supplements that will increase your stamina and sense of well being. If there is no joy in your life except what is brought on by an alcohol high, you need spiritual peace with your CREATOR and constant joy will be a by-product.

Even though a person who craves alcohol may stop drinking alcohol by sheer will power, the offending chemicals will stay in the brain unless removed by this method. If the offending chemicals are not removed, the craving will remain for YEARS. I personally had an uncle who was an alcoholic, but joined

172

AA. He told me YEARS after he totally quit drinking that every moment of every day he craved alcohol, but by sheer personal will power he decided he would never drink again because of the great suffering he caused every one around him when he was drunk. During this time of abstinence, HE HAND DUG AN IN-GROUND SWIMMING POOL FOR HIS FAMILY and HAND BUILT AND PERSONALLY MANAGED A FAMILY RESTAURANT just to keep himself busy and off alcohol. How I wish he knew this information before he died that Dr. Clark has recently discovered!!

To insure the beryllium does not come in contact with you, there are several precautions you can take. Remove all hurricane or antique lamps from the home. Washing does not remove the chemical. Remove all stored paints, thinners, solvents, lighters including barbecue lighters from the home. They can be stored in an out building NOT attached to the home. Switch to all electric heating. The garage door should be permanently sealed off from the rest of the house or the garage itself should be closed and never used again to store the car, lawnmower, small engine lawn or garden tools or machines, or chemicals mentioned above. People with alcoholic cravings should never work as a painter, near or with automotive products, or in a dry cleaning business (independent painters have the highest percentage of alcoholism of any profession!!!) The pathways in the brain opened and maintained by the beryllium will be filled quickly again, even after the beryllium is removed, if the beryllium is ever present in the future.

How is it that some people can have a drink and not even think about alcohol for months and others think about it constantly and must have it on a daily basis? The answer has been found. Only those who have the beryllium and ergot are "addicted". Although taking in alcohol at anytime is not health building for anyone, the person who can just have one glass of wine and never care if he has another alcoholic drink again or not does not have the ergot/beryllium problem-THAT IS WHY THEY CAN TAKE OR LEAVE ALCOHOL. It is only when the ergot/beryllium is present that the craving is there.

FACTS ABOUT ALCOHOL

Every single time you consume alcohol, you kill off some brain cells.

Red wine keeps down blood fats, but so does red grape juice (and purple and white grape juice, also).

THERE IS ABSOLUTE PROOF THAT DRINKING ALCOHOL WHILE PREGNANT CAN PERMANENTLY DAMAGE YOUR UNBORN CHILD!

Beer contains brewer's yeast, a substance very high in energy producing B-complex vitamins. If the diet is very low in B-complex vitamins because few whole grains or greens are eaten or if the diet is very high in fats or sugars, there will be a craving for B-complex vitamins. Some people get their only and greatest dose of these from beer. Therefore, they associate a calming of the nerves and energy boost from the B-complex vitamins in beer while getting a very dangerous dose each of alcohol and ergot at the same time. They would be much better off taking a high potency B-complex tablet (B-75 or B-100) with every meal and leaving the mold and alcohol laced beer alone.

Even small amounts of alcohol affect the throat, liver, brain, pancreas, duodenum, and central nervous system for the worse. It suppresses the immune system and affects the metabolic chemical reactions IN EVERY SINGLE CELL IN THE BODY. Daily consumption of alcohol shortens the life 10 to 15 years or more.

The liver can regenerate cells if part of the liver is removed, but if the cells are damaged by alcohol consumption, those cells can not reproduce.

Alcoholics have a much higher rate of mouth, throat, stomach, liver, colon, and breast cancer. They also have higher blood pressure, lower testosterone levels (decreased sex drive), higher blood vessel dilation (rosy skin), higher rates of congestive heart failure, more miscarriages, and more birth defects in their children than can be found in the non-drinking population.

If you can not go 24 hours without craving alcohol or thinking about it constantly, or looking forward to the next time you can get an alcoholic drink, you have an alcohol craving caused by the above factors. You are only free of it if not having another drink would never bother you at all. Buy the non-harmful supplements listed here and start on the road to being craving free and much healthier. If you are diligent in taking the supplements, you will start not craving the alcohol in a very short time- in a few days or in 2 or 3 weeks.

HOW TO GET THE ENERGY OF AN ALCOHOLIC HIGH WITHOUT ALCOHOL

When your energy sags, drink 100% orange juice, 100% blue grape juice, fresh carrot juice, ginger juice in small amounts or fresh parsley juice. These give you instant and long term energy and build up your health at the same time. Drinking these several times a day will keep blood sugar levels constant. Using these is much more effective than taking in carbonated, sugar-laden, caffeine loaded soft drinks AND their effects last much longer AND there are no bad side effects from them.

Raw sunflower seeds have every nutrient known to man except Vitamin C. If your energy is dropping, eat these to provide everything your body needs to get going strong again.

People who are under stress or who work long, hard hours can use B-complex vitamins (B-75 or B-100) many times a day to keep their energy levels up with no harmful side effects. If you take in too much, you just eliminate the excess through the urine. Take one tablet 3 to 8 times a day, as needed.

RELIEF FOR THE ADDICTION

For those of you who have fought for great periods of time against the craving, the time for remorse, guilt, sorrow, regret, hopelessness, self conflict, and compromised consciences is over. The problem is purely chemical and can be corrected in a relatively short period of time.

CHAPTER 39

STOP SMOKING NATURALLY

Whatever you have to do, just do it. There is not one good healthy thing that comes out of smoking or chewing tobacco. There are so many good options...

Get Peelu Smoker's Gum.

When you decide to stop, whenever you feel the need for a cigarette, eat a small peeled carrot, celery, or a small handful of sunflower seeds. Sunflower seeds kill cravings.

Take Green Vibrance, Perfect Food, or Buried Treasure VM 100 every morning and at lunchtime. Both of these kill cravings of any kind.

Get the nicotine gum if you have to.

Get the incremental nicotine patch if you have to.

Chew one piece of natural black licorice (Black Scottie dogs!) when the craving hits.

Drink Essiac or Flor-Essence tea every time a craving hits.

Take B-100 tablets every hour on the hour during the first week or so. It steadies the nerves. Carry a small bottle of them in your pocket every day.

Take 10,000 mgs. ester, buffered vitamin C throughout the day to detoxify.

Ying's Tea Capsules has helped some people be tobacco craving free in ONE DAY.

Independence Control Formula P-1 is another herbal formula that works for many.

Nicoban or SmokeRX are 2 more excellent formulas to kill the cravings and fill in the deficiencies caused by former smoking.

Just do whatever needs to be done to STOP SMOKING!!

CHAPTER 40

THE PERFECT ATHLETE'S DIET ???

The number one cause of death in retired athletes is colon cancer.

Why is this?

Athletes are told by uninformed trainers that to build and maintain muscle they must eat large quantities of protein, usually in the form of a highly concentrated protein powder in addition to large quantities of meat. They are told to do this without including generous amounts of green vegetables, fruits, and whole grains in the diet. This is deadly.

The human body produces daily enough hydrochloric acid and digestive enzymes to digest about 60 grams of protein. If much more than that is consumed, it passes through the body undigested. Once the undigested protein gets to the colon, it starts fermenting or going through a process called putrefaction then on to a much more serious condition called autointoxication. Because very few fiber foods are eaten by athletes, there is nothing to help push this undigested food mass through the intestines. This mass, which by this time is the consistency of cement or concrete, can literally sit there in the intestines for days, putrefying, putting off toxins and wastes that then pass through and even stay lodged in the intestinal wall (this is autointoxication). If it passes through the wall, it enters the blood stream where it can cause later muscle aches, dizziness, headaches, general weakness, and general malaise (you just do not feel well). The toxins that lodge in the intestinal wall form a perfect environment for cancer to grow. Years of continually eating a "perfect" athlete's diet will eventually cause colon cancer.

If the undigested protein is in the stomach, unmoved, it can cause nausea and pain. The mass just sitting in the intestine can cause pain, cramping in the lower bowel area (because the normal peristalsis or muscular contraction of the intestine is no match to this concrete-like mass), as well as the by-product of fermentation, continual intestinal gas.

Sometimes a very painful pain is felt in the end of the anus (most people describe this pain as the most distressing pain they have ever felt- it is very difficult to deal with, especially if you are on the job). This cramp is from the muscles trying to move this very hard mass and from the pressure of the mass on the nerve endings near the ending sphincter muscle of the anus. It can also be from a parasite changing positions as it feeding off this putrefying mass.

HOW TO UNDO THE DAMAGE, NATURALLY

Conventional medicine has no cure or pill for this condition. All doctors give are antacids to completely stop all digestion, a stool softener, and surgery to remove the damaged colon. None of these solve the condition or prevent it from reoccurring or progressing. If you want to totally restore the function of your intestines, there are measures you can take that are completely harmless. These will clean the intestine and the intestinal wall, rebuild the intestine where necessary, allow you to form and pass a comfortable stool, and maintain a sanitary, healthy digestive tract. You can be pain free in the matter of 3 to 10 days on this regimen. You can also have 2 to 3 effortless, odorless, and well-formed stools daily as a result of following this regimen, which will leave you with a relaxed, energetic feeling, and no pain. Here is how to do it---

Limit protein intake to around 60 grams daily.

Eat generous portions of green vegetables, raw (as in salads) or cooked (spinach, turnip greens, collards, kale,) and other vegetables such as carrots, sweet potatoes, baked potato, asparagus, celery, cabbage, broccoli, etc.

Eat fruits, but preferably non-citrus ones (apples, pears, bananas, grapes, berries, mango, papaya, pineapple, etc.)

If bread is eaten, never again eat white bread. Remember when you were a child how you used to squish a whole piece of white bread into one little sugar-cubed size square? All white flour products are worth nothing but for very good colon cloggers. Eat only whole grain breads. These contain many more nutrients, and the bran in the whole grains gently and continually cleans out your whole digestive system.

Follow the supplement regimen in the section BOWEL CONDITION CHECKLIST. These supplements will restore normal bowel function relatively quickly. Soon every day will be pain free.

Because undigested protein and deposited junk food may have been in the intestines for years, pockets may have formed in the intestines, making perfect homes for parasites and bacteria. Because of this I urge ALL CLIENTS WITH ANY BOWEL DISTURBANCE TO TAKE A 6 WEEK PARASITE CLEANSE. The flax fiber will eventually clean out the pockets and restore smooth elasticity to the intestinal wall. The parasite killing herbs will kill parasites in the intestinal wall and other organs, if they are present. (Parasites can feed quietly for years on undigested food in the intestine. The waste products of the parasites are also toxic. Sometimes the pain in the intestine is caused by the parasites themselves or their waste products.)

Taking these measures will restore normal bowel function and normal digestion. You will soon feel no discomfort in the lower bowel or stomach areas. You will have more energy, fewer headaches, fewer muscle aches, fewer cramps, less nausea, less intestinal gas, and fewer times of weakness.

You can really benefit by going on the Normal Bowel Function Restoration Diet in the next chapter FOR A WEEK OR TWO.

The first few days on the regimen may be difficult, but not everyone experiences this. You will be starting to move a large, undigested mass through approximately 22 feet of intestine that may be partially shrunken in size. Drink plenty of water and fruit juices (non-citrus, like 100% grape, apple, pineapple, mango, etc.) Hot peppermint tea with honey tames down the pain and discomfort. Massage any area where there is pain and apply heat to tender areas, if necessary. (Sometimes the diameter of the intestine shrinks down to pencil thin from faulty eating. Soon the intestine will stretch again to its proper size, but, at first, you may experience discomfort in the area. Every day the pain and discomfort should be less and less.) Take small rests lying down whenever possible. Keep warm. NO MATTER WHAT HAPPENS, KEEP TAKING THE RESTORATIVE SUPPLEMENTS. The supplements are not what are making you feel badly. It is the movement, finally, of the undigested mass that is making you feel badly. In a few days you will be feeling better. Take a 250 mgs. magnesium tablet to soften the stool and ease some of the pain. Never force feed yourself again.

CHAPTER 41

THE NORMAL BOWEL FUNCTION RESTORATION DIET

Using organic food is ALWAYS best.

Breakfast---

Stewed or baked apples, unsweetened applesauce, finely grated raw apple, no sweetening, Delicious or Golden Delicious apples are best.

Very ripe (yellow and spotted), raw, baked, broiled, or steamed bananas or ripe, baked plantains.

Lunch---

Yams, sweet potatoes, or Irish potatoes, baked, steamed, broiled in jacket- to be eaten without skin.

One or two steamed vegetables

If still hungry, a baked apple

No salt or butter.

Carrots, parsnips, turnips, squash, eggplant, tender string beans, tender okra, young peas are especially good. If condition is severe, pureeing may be necessary to eliminate large fibers. Red pepper (cayenne) may be sprinkled on vegetables.

Pureed soups containing only vegetables.

Dinner---

Same as lunch

Snacks---

Canned in its own juice fruit (peaches, pears, apricots), no sugar

Mashed, ripe mango, papaya, or avocado

100% fruit or vegetable juices - no sugars or colorings added

Water

Herbal teas

Proteins from the list PROTEINS FOR VEGETARIANS (Chapter 50) are the only proteins you may eat during this time of restoring bowel function, if you desire protein.

Bake, boil, broil, or steam your fruits and vegetables in glass or white Corning ware only.

This diet gives the digestive system time to calm down, lose inflammation and swelling, and start to repair. It may work in 1 to 3 weeks. Consistency is the key to returning to normal bowel functioning. Chew very well all food.

Puree or blend food in a blender if condition is severe. Organic baby food containing only the above ingredients may be eaten, also. Jars of organic baby food may be carried to work, etc. for snacks and emergency times of hunger.

Try not to snack. This gives the digestive system a chance to rest and repair between meals. Drink plenty of fluids between meals, but do not force liquids. Just drink when you are thirsty. Eat plenty of what is allowed at mealtimes. Take supplements first as they are your medicine and fill up afterward with allowed food. Do not over fill yourself. You will be surprised how fast you will be feeling better.

You should take any supplements in your particular regimen WITH (or at the same time as) your meal. Any enzymes should be taken especially with the meal.

CHAPTER 42

WHAT DO HERBS DO?

Every plant based food you eat is from an "herb". Most of the plant foods we eat most frequently are very watery herbs with a low nutritive content compared to most other plants. We consume regularly onions, celery, many types of lettuces, zucchini, yellow squash, string beans, cabbage family members like cauliflower, broccoli, rapini, Brussels sprouts, different types of cabbages, and broccolini, Swiss chard, tomatoes, cucumbers, mild radishes, parsley, etc. These have nutritive value, but low concentrations of medicinal qualities. These watery vegetable herbs usually have very little taste to them, but are mild in flavor. This is why it is easy and comfortable to repeatedly consume them. They are appealing to us because they have enough nutrients to take care of the daily housekeeping of a normally functioning, healthy body.

When you are sick, your body needs additional naturally occurring chemicals to deal with the many things that are disturbing your health we talked about at the beginning of this book. To correct these conditions, medicinal herbs are needed. These herbs are usually not very good tasting, but taste bitter because they contain VERY SPECIFIC chemicals needed by the body in very specific conditions. They are highly concentrated in these medicinal nutrients. You would not enjoy eating these herbs very frequently because of their very strong flavor. Your body would soon tire of them and reject them because they contain too many strong chemicals for your body to use constantly. This is why they are called medicinal herbs. They are to be used as medicine. Medicine is only needed when you are sick, and then you stop the medicine. They are reserved for just those times when you are sick.

An interesting fact about herbs is that you can take most herbs from all over the world and combine them in a tea, and no adverse reaction will happen. Try doing that with random conventional drug combinations! No, really, do NOT do that!

There are categories of herbs for every type of illness the human body can contract. There are colon cleansing herbs, laxative herbs, digestive aiding herbs, colon rebuilding and refurbishing herbs, herbs for the heart, liver, kidneys, and pancreas, antiviral herbs, antibacterial herbs, antifungal herbs, mold killing herbs, parasite killing herbs, herbs for muscles and broken bones, etc. These herbs can be used in very specific ways to bring health to the body after it is cleansed of harmful substances.

The regimens in the following chapters use very specific herbal combinations to accomplish very specific tasks. Taken a step at a time, you can heal your body of about anything!

There are many excellent books on the specific qualities and uses of herbs. The bible of herb books for North American herbs is BACK TO EDEN by Jethro Kloss.

There are cycles of enlightenment and use of the next "it" health food, herb, fruit, super food, or natural supplement as the years have passed. I feel the "next big thing" will be neem herb. It is so all encompassing in its uses, everyone should take it every day! For more information, go to www.ALLAB OUTNEEM.com.

Essential oils are the essences of medicinal herbs. These are the very strongest, fastest acting natural medicine available to mankind. The books HEALING OILS OF THE BIBLE and CHEMISTRY OF ESSENTIAL OILS MADE SIMPLE by David Stewart show the superiority and simplicity of the workings of essential oils in our bodies. The book THE ESSENTIAL LIFE is a great reference for the use of essential oils. I use them daily in many different applications. They work very fast to relieve much suffering quickly. Our Scriptural ancestors knew of their uses as they as mentioned about 1,000 times in Scripture!

CHAPTER 43

BASIC COMPREHENSIVE PARASITE CLEANSE

The following is a basic comprehensive parasite cleanse. It contains herbal combinations to kill parasites, bacteria, and viruses all at the same time. This regimen kills over 200 different types of possible parasites that can inhabit the human body from North America, Central America, South America, Europe, Southeast Asia, India, and Africa. This should be followed from 3 to 12 weeks depending on your symptoms. You will know parasites are gone when you have no reaction to the various elements of the program. You will feel perfect peace in your tissues and digestive tract once they are completely gone. Once you feel they are gone, go several days longer and then stop.

PARASITE CLEANSE CHART

PRODUCT	WHEN ARISING	BREAKFAST	LUNCH	DINNER	WHERE PURCHASED
PARATTHUNDER	6				WWW.WHITESAGELANDING.COM OR PURE PLANET PARASITE CLEANSE
NEEM CAPSULES	2		2	2	WWW.ALLABOUTNEEM.COM
HERBAL HEALER ACADEMY 500 PARTS PER MILLION COLLOIDAL SILVER		½ t.	½ t.	½ t.	WWW.HERBALHEALER.COM or www.vitacost.com
KYOLIC ODORLESS GARLIC #101 OR #102		2	2	2	WAL-MART or WWW.VITACOST.COM
COLONIX				½ SCOOP	WWW.DRNATURA.COM
BURIED TREASURE ACF		1 T.	1 T.	1 T.	WWW.VITACOST.COM
KLEARITEA				½ CUP	WWW.DRNATURA.COM
CO-ENZYME Q-10		3 TO 4 GRAMS			WWW.VITACOST.COM for 5 days
GARDEN OF LIFE RAW ENZYMES		1 OR 2	1 OR 2	1 OR 2	WWW.VITACOST.COM
CARROT/PARSLEY JUICE					2 CUPS DAILY
RAW PROBIOTICS BY GARDEN OF LIFE VAGINAL CARE		6/2		2	WWW.VITACOST.COM 6 THE FIRST DAY,2 THEREAFTER

PARASITE CLEANSE DIET

During the time of the Parasite Cleanse (at least 3 weeks), you should eat these foods as frequently as possible, as they are known to kill parasites also, incorporating them into your diet every day if possible...

Cucumbers, fennel seeds, parsley, cilantro, raw pumpkin seeds, carrots, carrot/parsley juice, pomegranate juice, Xango juice. Many people make a daily salad of the vegetables.

DO NOT EAT ANY MEAT, DAIRY, EGGS, OR FRESH FISH DURING THIS PARASITE CLEANSE. THIS IS TO INSURE YOU DO NOT GET REINFECTED DURING THIS TIME PERIOD. EAT A VEGAN DIET WITH HUMMUS, CHIA, MILLET, LENTILS, QUINOA, AND MANY KINDS OF VEGETABLES, LOW SUGAR FRUITS, NUTS, AND SEEDS AS YOUR MAINSTAY. MANY PEOPLE SAY THEY ARE FULL ON THE SUPPLEMENTS, JUICES, AND TEAS ALONE.

YOUR DIET SHOULD BE ORGANIC, DAIRY FREE, GLUTEN FREE, AND VEGAN FOR THIS TIME PERIOD.

This parasite cleanse contains natural parasite killing herbs and other natural agents known to kill parasites such as myrrh, golden seal, green black walnut hulls, wormwood, cloves, garlic, carrot, parsley, fennel, pomegranate, pumpkin seeds, parsley, carrots. If you make up your own parasite cleanse, it should contain as many of the above herbs as possible.

CHAPTER 44

HOW TO CURE YOURSELF OF CANCER

IT DOES NOT MATTER HOW BAD THE DISEASE IF YOU HAVE THE RIGHT MEDICINE!

An article I read recently quoted a coroner saying EVERY SINGLE BODY HE AUTOPSIED HAD CANCER GROWING IN IT, EVEN IF THE PERSON DID NOT EVEN DIE OF IT!!!!

Another recent article revealed that one in every four deaths in America is now caused by cancer.

Does anyone but me associate the word EPIDEMIC to these statistics??

With the BILLIONS of dollars spent on finding a cure in the past decades, WHY has there not been a cure discovered in conventional medicine research? One Stanford University researcher for AIDS says researchers live off research grants. They will research just about anything in order to keep getting research money. He says we should be able to trust researchers to do pure research and to seek out rock bottom scientific truths, but it just isn't true anymore. He says researchers will sometimes slant their research findings to favor the firm giving them the research money. Researchers also make their research so specific, such as looking for this enzyme or that amino acid to be the SOLE cause of a specific disease, that they ignore the MULTIPLE factors that set up a perfect environment for disease to proliferate and, then, never discover the real, associated causes. Another reason researchers do not quickly find a cure is that they elect to choose any of a million possibilities to research instead of finding those who have been cured of their disease and pinpointing common factors among them.

In the 1940's, Dr. Virginia Livingston-Wheeler decided to make her life's work a cure for cancer. In her research, she discovered that ALL the blood samples of ALL of her cancer patients had an acid-fast bacterium in them. She discovered this accidentally. This bacterium she named CRYPTOCIDES PROGENITOR ("deadly stalker"). Over time, she discovered an acid, abscisic acid, which would de-activate this bacterium. In other words, this acid is the antibiotic for this bacterium. In tests with people, chickens, and sheep, she could turn cancer on and off like a light switch, depending on the amounts of bacteria or acid she allowed them to have. She tested as many foods as she could for their abscisic acid content. In these tests, she found carrot juice, mango, avocado, very dark green leafy vegetables, and root vegetables had very high levels of the acid, with CARROT JUICE having the very highest amount per serving. She found ALL VEGETABLES have SOME abscisic acid in them. MOST animal products have very LITTLE abscisic acid. MOST VEGETABLES have very little of the specific bacteria in them. MOST animal products have A LOT of the specific bacteria in them.

She found that THE ENTIRE COMMERCIAL MEAT SUPPLY (in the many places she tested it across the USA) in the United States is contaminated with the bacteria. At this point, the USDA does not even acknowledge that the bacteria exists, let alone examine or test for it in USDA inspections.

There is more, but let's stop right here for a moment. We have heard of a coroner who says every dead person has cancer growing in him or her, bacteria that is in every cancer patient, and a meat supply loaded with the bacteria. At the same time, we have a population that eats lots of this bacteria laden meat and very little of the foods that kill off the bacteria in their bacteria-laden bodies. Does it now surprise you that so many people have cancer?

Here's the MORE. Dr. Livingston Wheeler also discovered that the bacterium manufactures, while in the body, a hormone that actually causes the rapid growth of cancer cells. This is a gonadotrophic hormone, which is the same hormone that is manufactured when an egg and sperm combine in the uterus to cause a baby to form in 9 months. If it only takes 9 months for a baby and all the tissue that accompanies a baby's growth (about 20 pounds) to form with this hormone as its engine, you can see how tumor tissue with this bacteria-produced hormone can grow VERY RAPIDLY.

DO NOT EAT SPROUTS! BUT DO EAT SHOOTS! Sprouts contain at the root tips this gonadotrophic hormone. It causes the root to grow cells very rapidly. So the seed plus the root should not be eaten. But the shoot of a sprout (the green part that grows above the soil) is very nutritious and safe! Eat shoots, not sprouts!

I know of cancer patients who started eating lots of sprouts who only progressed in the cancer faster! They should have eaten shoots instead!

Wait! There's EVEN MORE. She also discovered that the bacteria grow VERY RAPIDLY in the presence of sugar, as all bacteria do. High starch foods that break down into simple sugars also accelerate the growth of cancer. Now think about the VERY HIGH SUGAR CONTENT OF THE AMERICAN DIET.

Considering the high sugar and carbohydrate content of the American diet, and the high meat consumption that accompanies it, along with the VERY LOW OR NON-EXISTANT vegetable content of the American diet, you can see why so many people have cancer.

Dr. Hulda Clark discovered that in every cancer patient she tested, a parasite was found. This parasite produces, while in the body, viruses and bacteria, which are released into the tissues. When the parasite is killed through electric "zapping" and using herbal killing combinations, the viruses and bacteria eventually are killed off by a strong body or by adding strong herbal anti-virals and anti-bacterials. A weakened body may need help from herbal bacterial and viral killing preparations to finish and accelerate the cleansing.

SO, a parasite produces bacteria, which in turn produces a hormone that causes the rapid growth of cells in any part of the body, which we call CANCER !!!

As is well known, cancer is named by its location. Although you have heard of many types of cancer, it is really all the same disease, but just identified by where it is found. It appears that the cancer forms in any place the parasite or bacteria lands, no matter what type of tissue or location. It also appears that you may "kill" it off or remove it in one location (by surgery, chemotherapy, or radiation), but it will start growing in some other place if the body is not totally disinfected of it. The parasite and bacteria can travel in the blood or lymph system and lodge wherever there is a perfect environment for them to grow.

This is an aside, but there was a dentist in the 1970's who discovered that cancer could only grow in tissues that had been damaged in some way. A pocket forms at the damaged area. This pool in the circulation apparently forms a place for parasites and bacteria to stop and proliferate instead of being constantly moving and being flushed out of the system.

Back to Dr. Clark.... Dr. Clark also discovered that there is always a high concentration of propyl alcohol in the area where the cancer is found. She also found that the parasite that is in the cancer chain of growth grows very well in the propyl alcohol.

The most successful permanent eradication of cancer comes by killing off the parasite first, killing off the bacteria second (because it is continually manufactured by the parasite and will be present until the parasite is dead), dismantling the hormone, and then building up the body to clean out the residue, stopping the use of all propyl alcohol products, and, then shrinking the tumor tissue. Using this approach with my clients over the years as an herbalist, they have had great success in permanently overcoming cancer.

When I started researching the cause and cure for cancer, I realized many people over time have had successful regimens FOR THEIR TIME. Each of these had to deal IN THEIR TIME with an increasingly more complicated chemical environment. If we still just ate only organic foods and had no water, air, or environmental pollution, I think carrot juice and a vegetarian diet like Jethro Kloss used would still work. But things have changed and become increasingly more complex chemically inside and outside of our bodies.

Jethro Kloss could cure people of cancer with just carrot juice and a vegetarian diet in the late 1800's and early 1900's.

Dr. Max Gerson, in the 1940's, could cure people with carrot juice and liver injections.

Mr. Hoxsey, in the 1920's through the 1950's, could cure people of cancer with a combination of herbs and minerals.

Rene Caisse, RN, in the 1930's and 1940's, could cure people with a 4 herb combination shown to her by Ojibwa Indians in Canada.

Dr. Virginia Livingston Wheeler, in the 1960's through the 1980's, could cure people with a vegetarian diet and self injected autogenous vaccines.

All of these worked IN THEIR TIME. But now, we have a much more complicated chemical environment, and we have other aspects we did not have in those times.

We NOW ALSO have an INTERNATIONAL HEALTH ENVIRONMENT. We are exposed to many more parasites, viruses, bacteria, molds, fungi and chemical pollutants than EVER in human history because of international travel, unchecked immigrants, and from getting our foods from many, many foreign countries.

Therefore, to get back to good health, in the case of cancer or any disease, we have to confront ALL OF THESE ISSUES, as well as return to a TOTAL organic food supply.

INDIVIDUAL THINGS THAT HAVE CURED CANCER

Here is a list of individual things individual people have reported that has cured their cancer since cancer has been named "cancer". There is some overlapping as you will see with some of them. By making a regimen including many of these things, your likelihood of actually overcoming cancer is very great.

Selenium- 200 mcgs. daily

Adding garlic to a mostly organic vegan diet with very infrequent fins and scales fish and lots of dark green vegetables

Carrot juice daily

Carrot/parsley juice daily

Pancreatic enzymes daily - trypsin and chymotrypsin (Wobenzyme)

A total vegan diet with daily carrot juice

Essiac herbal formula daily

Flor-Essence herbal formula daily – similar to Essiac

Chaparral tea daily

A thorough herbal parasite cleanse

Mango and avocado eaten daily

Cod liver oil taken several times a day

Neem capsules taken daily

Asparagus – cooked, 2 times a day for 3-6 months

Organic purple grape juice fasting for 1 month (no other food!)

EpiCor

½ teaspoon of baking soda 2 times daily

Taking high CBD hemp oil daily

HERBS THAT KILL CANCER-

Red clover blossoms, burdock root, golden seal root, yellow dock root, blue violet leaves, powdered myrrh gum, echinacea, aloes, blue flag, gravel root, bloodroot (CANSEMA formula for skin cancer), dandelion, African cayenne, chickweed, rock rose, agrimony, Oregon grape root, and fo-ti in any combination taken as a tea or powdered in capsules.

CHAPTER 45

WHAT REALLY HAS BEEN PROVEN TO CAUSE CANCER???

From all the study I have done so far, it appears to me that this is what causes cancer –

These are all the findings, PROVEN AND REPEATABLE, which have been researched and proven consistent with cancer growth...

A PARASITE usually from MEAT or UNWASHED VEGETABLES or HOUSEHOLD PETS enters TISSUE sometimes PREVIOUSLY DAMAGED by physical force
in an environment of PROPYL ALCOHOL from FOODS and PERSONAL CARE PRODUCTS (which produces a cancer growth factor [ortho-phospho-tyrosine, along, with possibly, an epidermal growth factor and insulin-dependent growth factor]

Produces a BACTERIA (progenitor crypicides) that is smaller than most bacteria and has viral and fungal as well as bacterial qualities

Which produces an HUMAN CHORIONIC GONADOTROPHIN hormone (hCG) - which

Causes the rapid growth of cells we call cancer

Freon, copper, fiberglass, asbestos, mercury, lead, formaldehyde, and nickel accumulate in tissues and form non-malignant tumors. If the baby stages of the parasite reaches these propyl alcohol saturated tissues, cancer malignancy forms and then infection of bacteria sets in, then the hormone is produced and spurs RAPID growth.

INTERESTING FACTS RELATED TO CANCER

The highest sources of abscisic acid, in descending order, are- carrot juice, avocado, mango, any root vegetable, any green leafy vegetable, any vegetable.

The healthy human liver produces small amounts of abscisic acid. It produces enough to kill off small amounts of cryptocides progenitor under normal circumstances.

As an overtaxed liver slows its functions, it produces less abscisic acid. Remember, your liver has filtered out every HARMFUL, unwanted CHEMICAL that has entered your blood stream since it started functioning in your mother's womb.

When our main source of meat was wild origin or small homestead grown, the animals ate lots of uncontaminated green vegetation that killed off the bacteria in THEIR OWN BODIES. Now that animals are grown in feedlots, shoulder to shoulder in 6 inches of mud and many years' worth of manure containing the bacteria and increasing the possibility of contaminating each other by constant close contact, the frequency of cancer in the meat itself is greater. Add to this the fact that the feed lot animals are today fed mostly corn, hormones, and antibiotics and hardly ANY green vegetable matter to kill off the bacteria in their own bodies before being slaughtered to be food FOR YOU!

To produce chemically the same amount of abscisic acid as is in one 8 ounce glass of freshly prepared carrot juice and sell it in pill form would cost over $270.00 a pill!!

The typical farm diet of 75 years ago and previous to that consisted of organically grown greens (turnip, collard, and wilted lettuces), root vegetables (sweet potatoes, parsnips, turnips, rutabagas, and white potatoes), beans, and occasional meat—sometimes only once a week!! White sugar was reserved for very special and rare occasions. They had rare occurrences of cancer. They also used no propyl alcohol based personal care products (shampoo, hand lotion, deodorant, aftershave, shaving cream, perfume, hair conditioner, etc.) products back then.

The parasite that eventually produces cancer grows unchecked in tissues saturated in propyl alcohol substances. These substances include most commercially produced soaps, shampoos, hair styling aids, perfumes, after shaves, colognes, and some foods. (See list) These substances should be eliminated if cancer is to be totally conquered.

One area of China has the exact same diet (mostly vegetarian) as the rest of the general population of the country except they consume a lot of garlic there. RESEARCHERS IN THIS AREA COULD FIND NOT ONE INCIDENT OF CANCER!!! Garlic kills parasites, bacteria, yeasts, and viruses.

Yellow nutritional yeast kills cancer cells on contact.

Pancreatic enzymes trypsin and chymotrypsin start the death of cancer cells.

Cooked asparagus stops cancer cell growth.

Some people, but not all, have been cured of cancer by only adding selenium to their diet.

Some people, but not all, have been cured by adding cod liver oil to their diet.

THOUSANDS OF PEOPLE have cured themselves of cancer with the Essiac or Flor-Essence or the Herbal Healer Academy 4 Herb Formulas which are all basically the same formula under different names.

Dr. Virginia Livingston Wheeler of the Livingston Wheeler Cancer and Immunological Clinic in San Diego, California said the bacterium has bacterial, fungal, and viral qualities. She said the researchers have argued for years how to classify it, knowing it exists, but suppressing its existence from the general public.

William Russell, researcher, in the 1930's, found cancer parasites in most tumors.

G. G. Plimer, around 1900, found parasitic bodies in about 90% of tumors he researched.

Peyton Rous found a cancer causing agent in poultry called the Rous virus, for which every commercial chicken is NOW vaccinated (Rous vaccine).

James Young (1900), John Nuzum (1920), Michael J. Scott (1925), Georges Mazet(1942),Wilhelm von Brehmer(1945), Irene C. Diller(1950), Stearn, Sturdivant, and Stearn (1935), and T. J. Glover(1940) all detected, and the latter 2 isolated, pleomorphic(many formed) bacteria in cancer tissues.

William Reich (around 1937) discovered the actual microbe that could produce cancer in the laboratory.

Royal Rife (around1931) built a super microscope that revealed the cancer microbe.

John E. Gregory (around1945) discovered the same virus (IT COULD BE LABELED A VIRUS OR BACTERIA AS IT HAS CHARACTERISITICS OF BOTH— LIKE THE PLATYPUS HAS CHARACTERISTICS OF DIFFERENT SPECIES) form in all cancer tissues.

Dr. Virginia Livingston Wheeler (during 1940-1990) discovered a cancer microbe that had bacterial, fungal, and viral qualities.

Around 1960, Florence B. Seibert isolated bacteria from tumors and blood of cancer patients.

About 1990, M. W. White discovered again what so many had beforehand found, the microbe associated with cancer.

For those of you who think a cause for cancer has not been found, you are being misled.

There have been many people who have cured others and themselves of cancer documented since the early 1900's. Many researchers have found many answers and many others have repeated their research, but the established medical community is not releasing the information to the public. If you would like to read just one suppression of vital information story, read the book, THE CONQUEST OF CANCER by Dr. Virginia Livingston Wheeler to see how her research was shelved repeatedly. And you can read how she cured thousands of people at her clinic in San Diego, CA.

If the government REALLY wants to know what cures cancer, they should open a website where anyone who has cured himself of doctor diagnosed cancer can tell what he did to cure himself. Out of that information can be drawn commonalities that can be studied. Until then, just use the recommendations in this book!

CANCER REGIMEN CHART

PRODUCT	WHEN ARISING	BREAKFAST	10:00 AM	LUNCH	3:00 PM	DINNER	BEFORE SLEEP	WHERE PURCHASED
PARATHUNDER	6							WWW.WHITESAGELANDING.COM OR PURE PLANET PARASITE CLEANSE
BARLEY MAX		1 T.		1 T.		1 T.		WWW.HAACRES.COM
BURIED TREASURE ACF		1 T.		1 T.		1 T.		WWW.VITACOST.COM
RM-10 (GARDEN OF LIFE)		2		2		2		WWW.VITACOST.COM
KYOLIC TABLETS OR CAPSULES #101 OR #102		2		2		2		WWW.VITACOST.COM
COLONIX				½ SCOOP				WWW.DRNATURA.COM
500 PPM COLLOIDAL SILVER FROM HERBAL HEALER ACADEMY		½ t.		½ t.		½ t.		WWW.HERBALHEALER.COM OR WWW.VITACOST.COM
CARROT/PARSLEY JUICE 3/1 OR 4/1 PLUS ½ t. BAKING SODA			1 CUP		1 CUP		1 CUP	
WOBENZYME		3						WWW.VITACOST.COM
GARDEN OF LIFE RAW ENZYMES		1 OR 2		1 OR 2		1 OR 2		WWW.VITACOST.COM 2 at every major meal
MINT CHLOROPHYLL LIQUID				1 T		1 T		
RAW PROBIOTICS BY GARDEN OF LIFE		6 THE FIRST DAY, THEN 3 A DAY						WWW.VITACOST.COM
DIM		200 MGS.						WWW.VITACOST.COM
BLACK BOX DAILY DETOX							1 CUP DAILY	WHOLE FOODS
SELENIUM		200 MCGS						WWW.VITACOST.COM
COROMEGA ORANGE		1 PAK						WWW.VITAMINSHOPPE.COM
ASPARAGUS		½ CAN				½ CAN		
4 HERB FORMULA TEA AND CAPSULES		2 caps	1 cup	2 caps	1 cup	2 caps		WWW.HERBALHEALER.COM
CO-ENZYME Q-10		4 GRAMS						WWW.VITACOST.COM-FOR 5 DAYS ONLY
NEEM CAPSULES		2/2					2/2	WWW.ALLABOUTNEEM.COM
ESTER, BUFFERED VITAMIN C		3,000 MGS.		3,000 MGS.			4,000 MGS.	WWW.VITACOST.COM
CBD OIL-1500 MGS		½ tsp.						
MSM		3,000 MGS						
GRAVIOLA		2 CAPS						

CHAPTER 46

BASIC REGIMEN TO CURE YOURSELF OF CANCER

The ABOVE is a regimen in chart form that you can follow to START addressing curing yourself of cancer. This is the basic regimen I use with my clients. I make adjustments for each client's particular set of health problems beyond cancer, but these are the basic elements of a sound natural cancer regimen. It addresses parasites, viruses and bacteria released from the dying parasites, the hormones involved in cancer cell growth, and the bacterial, viral, and fungal qualities of the cancer microbe, and mold infections. I have used this regimen with hundreds of people with great success.

I have had clients be cancer free within just 6 weeks on this regimen. However, I have also had clients die at week 1, 2, and 3, but it appears if the clients can make it to the 4th week, they can complete the curing of themselves. In other words, it appears if the cases where the patient is told to just to go home and die can make it to the fourth week, they have the recuperative power to continue on to complete healing. To be successful with a natural regimen, it appears that you have to have the recuperative time of about 4 weeks to turn it around. Of course, none of us knows how much time we have left on out own personal timetable. Only the Father in heaven knows that. Only a few have died within the first 3 weeks, but it has to be mentioned.

This regimen can also be used by those who would like a little "insurance" against future cancer that has not been discovered YET in their body. It will clean out any factors that may be setting up the conditions for future rapid cancer growth. Some do this cleanse for 3 to 6 weeks a year as "insurance".

I truly believe this is not the only herbal cure for cancer. There are so many herbs in so many different locales on earth that surely there are more cures for cancer specific to each climate. Jethro Kloss' book BACK TO EDEN lists many herbs found in just North America that in the past in its less polluted environment cured cancer alone or in combination with other herbs.

This regimen contains many elements that individuals have used SINGLY to cure themselves of cancer THROUGHOUT THE YEARS IN AN INCREASINGLY MORE COMPROMISED ENVIRONMENT. Using MANY OF THESE TOGETHER GIVES AN EVEN GREATER CHANCE OF TOTALLY OVERCOMING CANCER.

In the 1940's, Dr. Virginia Livingston Wheeler, working at Rutgers, took slides of all her cancer patients' blood. After dyeing them with an acid-fast dye, she discovered a new bacterium that was found in every slide. It was a bacteriological cousin to the bacteria that cause tuberculosis and leprosy.

Over time, she discovered an acid, abscisic acid, which deactivates the bacterium. In other words, this acid was the antibiotic for the bacterium. The acid and bacterium occur naturally in foods. She did experiments with chickens, people, and sheep. First, she infected them with the bacterium. They developed all sorts of manifestations of cancer. Then she would feed them foods high in the acid, and the cancer would go away. She could turn cancer on and off like a light switch depending on if she fed them with the acid or the bacterium contained in their foods.

She opened a clinic, The Livingston Wheeler Cancer and Immunological Clinic, in San Diego, CA, where they have over an 85% cure rate on ALL types of cancer, including those told to go home and die by their doctors.

Eat these foods high in the acid to avoid cancer—

Carrots, Avocado, Mango—CARROT JUICE WITH PARSLEY

Any green leafy vegetable—kale, collard, turnip, romaine, frisee

Any root vegetable—garlic, sweet potato, rutabaga, onion, carrot, turnip

Any orange, red, or yellow vegetable—tomato, yellow squash

Berries

DO NOT EAT SPROUTS OF ANY KIND AS THE GROWTH HORMONE IN THE ROOT TIPS IS THE SAME HORMONE THAT MAKES CANCER CELLS GROW VERY RAPIDLY!!!!

Use amaranth, millet, quinoa, seeds plus beans, seeds plus the mentioned grains products for complete protein.

Do NOT eat these foods high in the bacterium—

Meat

Poultry

Eggs

Dairy (cow)

No sugar in any form because it makes the bacterium multiply.

REMEMBER!

Dr. Livingston found the meatpacking, dairy, poultry, and egg production systems to be totally contaminated with the bacterium. The USDA does not even acknowledge that the bacterium exists, let alone test for it.

In the 1990's, Dr. Hulda Clark discovered that parasites bring and manufacture this bacterium in their bodies into your body. She discovered that by bioelectric treatments, you can kill SOME of the bacteria and parasites instantly (Her books telling of her discoveries and treatment are named THE CURE FOR ALL DISEASES, THE CURE FOR ALL CANCERS and THE CURE FOR ALL ADVANCED CANCERS). She also found that certain herbs will kill off ALL the parasites and its different stages over a short period of time. Rebuilding health after this treatment then takes about 2 months, if a strong herbal and nutritional program is followed. This, used in conjunction with Dr. Livingston's knowledge, brings dismissal of cancer and its effects in about 2 to 3 months. I have had clients declared by medical tests cancer free in as short a time as 6 weeks on this regimen.

Dr. Virginia Livingston Wheeler found that the bacterium that is always present in cancer growth has viral, bacterial, and fungal qualities. These must be addressed to fully conquer cancer. She also discovered that whenever there is malignant cancer growth, there is a gonadotrophic hormone driving the rapid growth of the cells. She also discovered that abscisic acid deactivates the bacterium just like an antibiotic does other bacteria.

Dr. Hulda Clark discovered that there is always a certain liver fluke present nearby in malignant cancer growth. She also discovered that the tissues where cancer proliferates are highly saturated with propyl alcohol.

CHAPTER 47

THE CANCER DIET

A simple vegan diet of organic vegetables, low sugar fruits, seeds, nuts, and juices is the best diet route to beating cancer. NO SPROUTS!

Your supplements and juices are your medicine and your food FIRST before any other food is taken at each meal. The first few days on the regimen you may not feel like eating much food, but appetite will return in a few days, and the supplements have plenty of nutrition to keep you going. When desiring to eat food, eat as much in each category you need to feel satisfied. Always organic!

UPON ARISING

7 (21 if on advanced regimen) herbal parasite caps or tabs (PARATHUNDER, PURE PLANET PARASITE CLEANSE, or other).

BREAKFAST

Supplements

Juice (carrot/parsley)

1 choice from vegetarian protein list, if desired

Nuts, seeds, and/or berries

LUNCH AND SUPPER (OR DINNER)

(noon and evening)

Supplements

Carrot/parsley juice

Chopped cilantro

1 choice from vegetarian protein list, if desired

1 or 2 steamed or baked vegetables, cooked in Corning ware, if desired

Large raw vegetable salad with carrots and avocado included, if desired

SNACKS AND SEASONINGS

Raw nuts and seeds, fresh, raw vegetables, herbal teas, 100% raw vegetable juices, ORGANIC V-8, raw or roasted nut butters (no peanut butter), Vega Sal, PINK SALT, apple cider vinegar, POMEGRANATE VINEGAR, olive oil, flaxseed oil, herbs, spices, mustard, organic canned tomato products (Muir Glen, etc.), frozen OR JAR lemon juice, cayenne, turmeric, parsley, chives, garlic, mild or medium organic hot Mexican food type sauce or salsa without sugar, vegetable chips (with non- hydrogenated oils). NO SPROUTS!!!! EVER!!!

CHAPTER 48

THE CANCER DIET RULES

Organically grown foods should be preferred over any other type

No sugar in any form

ABSOLUTELY NO SPROUTS OR SPROUTED ANYTHING

No artificial flavorings, artificial colors, chemical preservatives, herbicides, or pesticides

GRAINS

No grains in any form

EXCEPTION – millet, quinoa, amaranth, BUCKWHEAT, GLUTEN FREE OATS OR OATMEAL

VEGETABLES

Baked, steamed, juiced, or raw. Cooked in Corning ware or clear glass only. Soups may be made of choices on list. Gumbo combinations can be made adding choices from protein list.

AVOCADO, CARROTS, AND ASPARAGUS (should be used every day), sweet potato, string beans, potato, rutabaga, turnip, parsnip, carrot, onion, garlic, leeks, chives, cilantro, beet, fennel, greens (turnip, spinach, kale, collard, rape, romaine, parsley, watercress, frisee, rapini, broccolini, escarole, dark, green and red lettuces, etc.), any salad vegetable, any green vegetable, any orange vegetable, any yellow vegetable, any red vegetable, any purple vegetable, any root vegetable, tomato, celery. Lentils, soybeans, black beans, fava beans, lima beans, kidney beans, garbanzo beans (chick peas), and kidney beans ONLY in the dried bean category. Any seed or nut. NO SPROUTS!!!

FRUITS

You must limit your fruit choices to these low sugar varieties. Berries are the best. Fresh, frozen, baked, stewed, juiced, or canned in juices ONLY.

MANGO (should be used EVERY day), SOURSOP, blueberries, raspberries, pineapple, strawberries, gooseberries, pomegranate, noni, gogi, mangosteen, lemon, peaches, passion fruit, apricots, peaches, elderberries, acai, pears, papaya, guava, lemon, lime, nectarine, TANGERINES, marionberries, cherries.

CHAPTER 49

PROPYL ALCOHOL PRODUCTS AND CANCER

Because there is an association between cancer growth and the concentrations of PROPYL ALCOHOL products in the tissues, if you have diagnosed cancer, you should avoid all products containing any PROPYL ingredients. This is found in almost every personal product on the market, such as soaps, deodorants, shampoos, creams, etc. LOOK FOR THE WORDS PROPANOL, ISOPROPANOL, ISOPROPYL ALCOHOL, any PROPYL suffix or prefix, and RUBBING ALCOHOL on the labels.

Propyl products will not GIVE you cancer. If the liver fluke causing cancer is present, propyl products will accelerate and protect the growth of cancer.

Substitute products for propyl products for cancer patients--

20 Mule Team Borax and washing soda can be used for washing about everything.

Apple cider vinegar, lemon juice, orange oil, soapnut, grapefruit oil, ammonia, and baking soda can be used to clean just about anything, as well as disinfect things.

ACCEPTABLE PRODUCTS

Always check and later recheck labels as product ingredients change as "improvements" are made to products............

The Besorah Seed products-www.allaboutneem.com

TERRESSENTIALS is the safest and best

Most Burt's Bees products

Most Tom's of Maine products

Most Aubrey products

Some Desert Essence products

Most 100% Pure brand products

Miessence

OTHER PROPYL POLLUTED PRODUCTS

(THESE INCLUDE MOST HEALTH FOOD STORE BRANDS AS WELL)===

SHAMPOO

HAIR SPRAY, MOUSSE, GELS

COLD CEREALS PRE-PACKAGED

COSMETICS, LIPSTICK, EYELINER, AND MASCARA ARE THE WORST!

MOUTHWASH

DECAF COFFEE, POSTUM, PRE-PACKAGED HERB TEA BLENDS

BOTTLED WATER IN PLASTIC

RUBBING ALCOHOL

WHITE SUGAR

ALL SHAVING SUPPLIES INCLUDING AFTERSHAVE

CARBONATED BEVERAGES

STORE BOUGHT FRUIT JUICES

CHAPTER 50

PROTEIN FOR VEGETARIANS LIST

I HAVE FOUND MY CLIENTS HAVE A MUCH GREATER CHANCE OF TOTALLY
OVERCOMING THEIR HEALTH PROBLEM IF THEY EAT A VEGAN DIET
WHILE TREATING THEMSELVES. AND THE MORE RAW ORGANIC
VEGETABLES THEY EAT, THE BETTER.

When you stop eating animal based protein for the duration of a parasite
cleanse, cancer regimen, AIDS or HIV+ regimen to avoid recontaminating
yourself from parasites, you still need complete protein. You need 22 essential
amino acids to rebuild body tissues. The following gives you ideas of how to get
complete protein without eating animal based protein. The book DIET FOR A
SMALL PLANET by Frances Moore Lappe is still the Bible of food combining to
get complete protein.

You may use any of these except those specified differently. Using soy-less
products is definitely preferable if you have other choices available.

The best healing diet is an organic diet of raw, fresh vegetables, low sugar
fruits, nuts, seeds, some whole grains fixed in a simple manner. Because some
people have a busy schedule working away from the home, this list below has
suggestions for fix-it-quickly meal elements.

Combining a bean and a grain at the same meal will yield complete protein.

Combining a seed and a grain at the same meal will yield complete protein.

COMPLETE PROTEIN SOURCES

Amaranth, buckwheat, hempseed, spirulina, hummus, quinoa, and millet are stand alone vegetable sources of complete protein. These sources are also gluten free.

Hemp milk (with no added sugars, if on cancer diet)

PROTEIN POWDERS

Amazing Meal

Hemp protein powder

IncaMeal

Most organic vegan protein powders

Organifi protein powder

BURGERS

Sunshine Burgers - many different flavors

Many new sources are coming on the market all the time. They should be organic and vegan. Any totally organic, vegan product that contains no sugar, artificial flavorings and colorings, or chemical preservatives (and starches or carbohydrate and sugars, if on the cancer diet).

There is some evidence that some of the soy based meat substitutes may have excitotoxins and extra estrogens for some people. If you feel this may be your case, use the non-soy products listed here. Eliminating soy products completely from your diet gives you an even better chance of overcoming cancer completely!

This list gives a good variety of choices for meat substitutes that contain complete protein that is the same complete protein as that in meat products.

CHAPTER 51

HOW TO CURE YOURSELF OF HIV+ STATUS AND AIDS
BRINGING YOU TO "VIRUS UNDETECTABLE" STATU

AIDS is an especially fearful condition for some right now because it seems in spite of all the research and drugs in use against it, nothing has been discovered by conventional drug-driven medicine that will restore the health of the patient and completely eradicate the virus from his or her system. The prognosis was 18 months in the 1980's. It was 25 years in 2010 because of some of the drugs now available, but they the patients never achieve "virus undetectable" status without the drugs.

It is relatively easy to overcome HIV status or even AIDS using an all-natural approach. It does appear, although, to take approximately 2 to 4 weeks MINIMUM to reverse the condition using an all-natural, herbal approach. Obviously, the patient must have this amount of time on their personal timetable of life to reverse the condition.

There are many conditions to consider when attempting to bring the patient to virus undetectable status.

The AIDS patient almost always has multiple parasitic, bacterial, as well as sometimes, multiple viral, mold, and fungal infections. These all can be dealt with by taking several comprehensive herbal anti-virals, anti-biotics, anti-fungals, and anti-helmetics (parasite killing).

Because the AIDS patient often has a lifestyle that entails frequent intimate, sexual contact with many people, this increases his or her possibility of cross infection without the time period of overcoming each infection (whether it be parasitic, bacterial, viral, mold, or fungal) individually. Therefore, the AIDS or HIV patient must stop all risky sexual activity in order to insure full recovery.

THE FOLLOWING DISCUSSION MAY NOT BE FOR EVERYONE, BUT IT MUST BE ADDRESSED BY SEXUALLY ACTIVE CLIENTS........

Since it is known that HIV/AIDS is spread through body fluids, any exchange on any level should be considered dangerous and have the potential for maintaining and prolonging the HIV/AIDS infection. Anal sex is especially dangerous as any ejaculated semen into the rectum is immediately and in its undigested state absorbed by the lower intestine and carried by the bloodstream to every part of the body. Oral sex is also dangerous as semen in the digestive tract is absorbed into the small intestine with its deadly contents. And vaginal discharge in the digestive tract is equally as dangerous.

The AIDS patient often is malnourished. He or she needs to be totally saturated with every nutrient to make an attempt to overcome the condition. He or she must eliminate all animal based foods for the duration of the disinfection program to also insure there is no re-infection of parasites and accompanying viruses, bacteria, and fungi. Ample vegetarian protein should be included in the diet as well as plenty of green vegetables and, in time, some fruits.

The patient may be so weak, he or she may need help preparing juices, tea, food, and supplements at first until he or she is stronger. This could be the job of a loving friend, relative, church or family group. Any one helping the patient should follow proper sanitary procedures with washing hands frequently being top priority.

The patient may be hospitalized. The caring team needs to be willing, aware, educated, and "on the same page" in the knowledge of the natural care treatment plan and regimen in the care of the patient.

Natural Herbal Therapy assumes no responsibility in the out care of anyone seeking to use and follow suggested treatments. Although the treatment has proven successful through use, there are so many uncontrolled variables that can happen or that cannot be detected. The supplements used in the regimen are harmless and body nourishing.

If the patient is on a feeding tube, the tablet form supplements can be powdered or capsule contents emptied and mixed with the teas and juices. Care should be taken that the mixture is fluid enough NOT to clog the tube.

Dr. Hulda Clarke has discovered an association between HIV, AIDS, and the chemical pollutant benzene and the intestinal fluke. The program you will be following will rid you of the fluke, but it will be your responsibility to endeavor to rid your body, home, and food supply of the benzene-laden products.

In the regimen you will be using, the steps proceed as follows-

Parasite cleansing - the intestinal fluke must be killed in order to stop the production of the virus associated with this condition (the fluke either produces or maintains the life or the production of the virus). An herbal powder known to kill approximately 200 different kinds of parasites will be used. Capsules and powder will be part of this cleansing. If this is the first parasite cleanse the patient has ever taken, it should continue for 3 months.

A viral, bacterial, fungal, and mold cleanse – since AIDS and HIV positive cases are known for having MULTIPLE infections, this MUST accompany the parasite cleansing. Also, as parasites die as the result of the parasite cleanse, they release stored bacteria and viruses that MUST IMMEDIATELY BE DEALT WITH OR INFECTIONS WILL INCREASE, INCREASING THE LOAD FOR THE IMMUNE SYSTEM.

To increase efficiency of the digestive tract to get maximum nutrition, a comprehensive digestive enzyme will be used until the patient is able to care for himself or herself, or for at least 6 weeks like Garden of Life Raw Enzymes.

To help rid the body of excess benzene and other heavy metals, a heavy metal cleanse will be introduced after a week or more on the parasite and microorganism cleanses like Toxinout or Daily Detox (black box) Tea.

To increase the immune capabilities, a multi-form acidophilus/bifidus probiotic formula will be used like Garden of Life Raw Probiotics for Women Vaginal Care- 38 forms.

Because the liver filters everything that enters the blood, a good functioning liver is top priority in any critical or chronic condition. Therefore, at the third week and every three weeks following for 3 months, a one day liver cleanse (flush) will be necessary.

A free form amino acid powder will be used for AT LEAST 4 weeks as the main protein source. It is easily and highly digestible, and it will take the place of meat, dairy, eggs, fish, and poultry (possible carriers of the parasite). Any organic vegan protein powder is only permissible. Plain organic unsweetened hemp milk, and plain organic whey powder are acceptable protein sources, also.

Because microorganisms can grow rapidly on any form of sugar, the diet must be free of any form of sugar except those forms in vegetables. The diet will consist of vegetables, teas, freshly made juices, free form amino acid powder, and later, some low sugar fruits.

Medicinal teas, juices, and supplements must be eaten before any other acceptable foods can be consumed at every meal.

INDIVIDUAL THINGS THAT HAVE CURED AIDS/HIV+

Here is a list of individual things that individuals have reported that have cured their AIDS or HIV+ status to the point of becoming "virus undetectable". By making a regimen of several or all of these things, your likelihood of actually overcoming AIDS is very great.

Selenium - 200 mcgs. daily

Pine Sol - I would not suggest this to anyone, but it must have been the pine oil in it!

Pine needle oil capsules

A parasite cleanse with antiviral herbs

I have had clients become "virus undetectable" as shown by blood test in as short a time as 4 weeks and as long a time as 18 months. But ALL THAT HAVE STAYED ON THE REGIMEN became "virus undetectable" eventually. The average time is about 8 weeks. You must be consistent and persistent. It will turn eventually if you are true to the principles shown in this book.

CHAPTER 52

BASIC REGIMEN TO CURE YOURSELF OF AIDS AND/OR HIV+ STATUS
BRINGING YOU TO "VIRUS UNDETECTABLE" STATUS

This is a good basic regimen to turn AIDS or HIV+ into "virus undetectable" status. I have had clients reverse this in as short as 4 weeks. I have had some who have been from Africa who probably have had an HIV+ status (and deep benzene absorption) since birth take 18 months to turn the testing to "virus undetectable". I know this regimen works. I have had many, many clients reverse their status. You just have to stay on it until the total cleansing and repair work is done. You must be consistent and do not give up. It will turn eventually if you keep on the regimen and follow the principles in this book.

Because most AIDS/HIV+ patients have multiple bacterial, multiple viral, multiple fungal and multiple parasite infections that are bringing their immune function down, this regimen addresses parasites, fungi, molds, viruses, bacteria, and chemical pollutants. Selenium deficiencies are always present in AIDS. Pine oil capsules disintegrate the virus itself when taken with the other elements of this regimen. When the immune system breaks down, all the codependent or symbiotic elements have to have their bonds broken by killing the stronger partner first. Then it is easier to get rid of the individual weaker partners that are left.

FOLLOW THE PARASITE DIET SHEET FOR 3 WEEKS OR LONGER AS YOU USE THIS SCHEDULE

AIDS AND HIV+REGIMEN

PRODUCT	WHEN ARISING	BREAKFAST	10:00 AM	LUNCH	3:00 PM	DINNER	BEFORE SLEEP	WHERE PURCHASED
PARATHUNDER	6							WWW.WHITESAGELANDING.COM OR PURE PLANET PARASITE CLEANSE
ESSIAC OR HERBAL HEALER ACADEMY 4 HERB FORMULA CAPSULES		1 CUP 4		1 CUP 4		1 CUP 4		WWW.PENNHERB.COM OR WWW.HERBALHEALER.COM
MSM		1500 MGS.				1500 MGS.		WWW.VITACOST.COM
BURIED TREASURE ACF		1 T		1 T		1 T		WWW.VITACOST.COM
HERBAL HEALER ACADEMY 500 PARTS PER MILLION COLLOIDAL SILVER		½ t		½ t		½ t		WWW.HERBALHEALER.COM OR VITACOST
KYOLIC GARLIC #101 OR #102		2		2		2		WWW.VITACOST.COM
B-100 COMPLEX TABLETS		1	1	1	1	1	1	WAL-MART OR WWW.VITACOST.COM
SELENIUM		200 MCGS.						WAL-MART OR WWW.VITACOST.COM
CARROT/PARSLEY JUICE			1 CUP		1 CUP			
NEEM CAPSULES		2		2		2		WWW.ALLABOUTNEEM.COM
ESTER, BUFFERED VITAMIN C		3,000 mgs		3,000 mgs		4,000 mgs		WWW.VITACOST.COM
GARDEN OF LIFE RAW ENZYMES		1 or 2		1 or 2		1 or 2		WWW.VITACOST.COM
GARDEN OF LIFE RM-10		6						WWW.VITACOST.COM
PINE OIL CAPSULES		2		2		2		WWW.PINE-HEALTH.COM
RAW PROBIOTICS BY GARDEN OF LIFE VAGINAL CARE		6/2						WWW.VITACOST.COM
CO-ENZYME Q-10		4 GRAMS						WWW.VITACOST.COM FOR 7 DAYS ONLY
ZINC GLUCONATE				50 Mgs				WWW.VITACOST.COM

CHAPTER 53

BENZENE POLLUTED PRODUCTS TO AVOID FOR HIV+/AIDS

There is an association between AIDS and benzene in the tissues. In most wells
in Africa where water is pumped up by a benzene producing petroleum run
motor, there is a higher occurrence of AIDS and HIV+ in the people using the
water from the wells than in non-benzene containing wells.

FLAVORED FOODS such as yogurt, Jell-o, candies, throat lozenges, store-
bought cookies, cakes

COOKING OIL AND SHORTENING (use only organic olive oil, coconut oil, and
butter)

BOTTLED WATER AND BOTTLED FRUIT JUICE whether distilled, spring,
mineral, or brand name

PACKAGED COLD CEREAL including granola and health brands

TOOTHPASTE including health brands

CHEWING GUM

ICE CREAM AND FROZEN YOGURT

ALL VASELINE PRODUCTS including Noxzema, Vick's, Lip Therapy, Chapstick,
and hand cleaners

RICE CAKES including plain ones

PERSONAL LUBRICANTS AND LUBRICATED CONDOMS

BAKING SODA AND CORNSTARCH

SOAPS, HAND CREAMS, SKIN CREAMS, MOISTURIZERS

FLAVORED PET FOODS FOR BOTH DOGS AND CATS

BIRD FOOD MADE INTO CAKES

Others may be added as discoveries continue.

CHAPTER 54

WHAT GAY AND BISEXUAL MEN SHOULD KNOW THAT NO ONE IS TELLING THEM

This may or may not apply to you, but if it does, you should know this!!!

Every time a man has an ejaculation, a large quantity of zinc is lost. Zinc is one of the most important building blocks of the immune system. The more frequent the ejaculations, the lower the zinc level in the body. The normal replacement time of zinc to keep the zinc level constant for an healthy immune system is an ejaculation approximately once every week and an half. The lower the zinc level, the weaker the immune system. This fact is essential to understand in overcoming HIV/AIDS status.

The lower intestine absorbs water and substances from any fluid introduced into it and puts those substances directly into the bloodstream. It normally absorbs water and nutrients from the digested food mass constantly passing through it. This is one of its jobs in the human body. Introducing any substance that is undigested is very dangerous and is like taking a direct transfusion of the substance. This, in itself, can be deadly because the bloodstream is set up to accept only fully digested substances. Semen and its components introduced into the lower intestine are absorbed by the intestine. This would include any viruses or bacteria that may be in the semen, as can be the case in HIV/AIDS or any infectious microorganism.

Any undigested proteins (such as are in semen) introduced into the lower intestine and forced into its tissues, begin a process called autointoxication. These undigested proteins settle into the intestinal wall and are perfect food for parasites, viruses, and other microorganisms. Weaknesses, cracks, cuts, fissures, or pockets formed by constant strain, friction, stretching, and the high powered forces of ejaculations, fisting, ballooning, or rubbing are perfect habitats for these offending organisms to multiply. Autointoxication is the first step in the progress of colon cancer.

The lower intestine is full of waste products from digestion such as bacteria, viruses, molds, fungus, parasites, pollutant chemicals, etc. Another one of its jobs in the human body is to protect and preserve the human body for prolonged life by transporting these life-threatening things OUT of the human body. When the delicate tissues of the lower intestine are broken by stretching, strain, fisting, ballooning, the high powered forces of ejaculations, rubbing, or friction, etc., these microorganisms are rubbed into the cracks, cuts, and fissures and are also directly transferred to the bloodstream.

The male penis at its head has a ridge where, circumcised or uncircumcised, bacteria accumulate. When these bacteria are introduced into the rectum, they also are directly absorbed into the blood stream. There is more bacteria accumulation under the skin of an uncircumcised penis than at the ridge of a circumcised penis. Whenever masturbation occurs, any bacteria on hands or penis near the opening of the penis can go up to the prostate and cause infection and inflammation.

If there is multiple partner contact without thorough washing in between contacts, any, or possibly all, of these above mentioned conditions may infect a gay or bisexual man AND ALL HIS SUBSEQUENT PARTNERS with multiple bacterial, viral, molds, fungal, parasitic, or chemical pollutant microorganisms which severely heighten the immune system load and lower immune system efficiency. Most HIV/AIDS patients have MULTIPLE viral, bacterial, fungal, mold, and parasitic infections from contact and cumulative infections from many partners.

ON THE OTHER HAND—

The female vagina is naturally clean, sterile, stretches easily and recovers from stretching rapidly, is constantly flushing itself out with sterile mucus, has no direct contact with the blood stream or fecal waste materials, but only a pathway to receive sperm and form babies, THE REAL PURPOSE OF SEXUAL INTERCOURSE.

CHAPTER 55

THE SCRIPTURES, YOUR SEXUAL LIFE, AND YOUR HEALTH- BLESSINGS AND CURSINGS

Just like the foods you put in your body matter, what goes in your body and How you handle your body SEXUALLY is very important and can impact whether you live or die, become healthy or continue in illness. There are ways that the body is to be used and the Bible also is very clear about how the body is not to be used, sexually.

The Creator created your body to be used in a specific way for specific functions. It is very popular these days to promote the sexual misuse of the body. In fact, talking about proper use of the body and proper sexual behaviour from a sin and health standpoint has become very rare, even in the churches.

The Bible speaks in Ephesians about not even speaking about things done in secret, referring to sexual sins. Very sincere people are very sincerely deceived in this area at this time in history. I feel it necessary to speak briefly about it as it pertains to your personal health.

Ephesians 5:3-12 KJV- But fornication, and all uncleanness, or covetousness, let it not be once named among you, as becometh saints; 4 Neither filthiness, nor foolish talking, nor jesting, which are not convenient: but rather giving of thanks. 5 For this ye know, that no whoremonger, nor unclean person, nor covetous man, who is an idolater, hath any inheritance in the kingdom of Messiah and of the Creator. 6 Let no man deceive you with vain words: for because of these things cometh the wrath of the Creator upon the children of disobedience. 7 Be not ye therefore partakers with them. 8 For ye were sometimes darkness, but now [are ye] light in the Creator: walk as children of light: 9 (For the fruit of the Spirit [is] in all goodness and righteousness and truth;) 10 Proving what is acceptable unto the Creator. 11 And have no fellowship with the unfruitful works of darkness, but rather reprove [them]. 12 For it is a shame even to speak of those things which are done of them in secret.

In everything we DO and THINK, there is a spiritual aspect to it as well as a physical aspect to it. Both intertwine in our heavenly Father's eyes as is so plainly taught in the blessings and cursings in Deuteronomy 27-30.

If you are serious about healing your body, you cannot do one thing that is healing and yet continue to engage in destructive behavior and expect optimal health. The Bible teaches us to avoid the unnatural use of our bodies- Romans 1:26. These are conducts that MUST be avoided both to honor the Creator and help your body reap blessings. A person can eat all organic foods to try and heal, but if they engage in deviant sexual conduct, they are sabotaging their body's immune system's ability to respond to threats. Our Creator is not mocked by our rebellious, unholy, unlawful behaviour. What we do sexually affects us physically and spiritually. Romans 1

The ONLY sexual expression that is sanctioned by the Creator to bring blessings and not curses is a certain act in marriage between one natural born man and one natural born woman in a monogamous marriage that has no sodomy, no fantasy, and no pornography.

1 Corinthians 6:19-20 - Flee from sexual immorality. Every other sin a person commits is outside the body, but the sexually immoral person sins AGAINST HIS OWN BODY. Or do you not know that your body is the temple of the Holy Spirit within you, whom you have from the Creator? You are not your own, for you were bought with a price. So glorify the Creator in your body.

Again, the Creator is not mocked when the body is used immorally. Deviant sexual behaviour brings curses, not blessings.

Many diseases and conditions, and certainly sexually transmitted diseases, are spread person to person by the body fluids urine, saliva, semen, vaginal fluid, and blood. These fluids can contain viruses, bacteria, molds, fungi, and parasites. Taking any of these wrongly by mouth, or vaginally, or rectally can cause horrible health problems, some even produce death.

We all know that when we have a bowel movement, that it comes mostly from food that we placed in our mouth, which was clean and safe, and ends up coming out the other end of our digestive tube as something filled with bacteria that can make someone so sick that they die if accidentally consumed. Cholera, polio, and e coli, for example, are all passed in the stool to others who accidentally got some in their water. Feces are not to be taken into the body in any fashion, but to be put away from the body, washed away from the body, and to be earth buried. Deuteronomy 23:13

The Bible speaks about the unnatural use of the body in Romans 1:26. There are many ways to use the body unnaturally. That means there must be a natural use of the body in sexual activity. This natural use of the body in sexual activity produces children, intimacy between a man and a woman dedicated people attended by personal shared pleasure, relaxation, and personal bonding with the produced hormone oxytocin that releases during sexual contact, birth, and breastfeeding. This hormone is also known as the "love" hormone. Married intimacy should be between a man and a woman caring for each other who already feel close and have resolved and talked and prayed through any hurts.

The following practices are deviant and destructive sexual acts and, while the culture may promote them as normal and okay, they are damaging to your body and spirit and will undermine and harm you and your health in many ways. If you want to avoid CURSES and reap BLESSINGS in the health area of your life, you must avoid these deviant sexual practices. Many of them originated as forms of pagan worship to demon gods. Those seeking to be obedient to the Heavenly Father need to have no part of them.

These deviant sexual practices cause many diseases by lowering the immune system or placing pathogens where they can attack the body. For example, almost all cervical cancer, anal cancer, and throat cancer are caused by Human Papilloma Virus (HPV), a sexually transmitted viral disease.

DEVIANT SEXUAL PRACTICES TO AVOID

FORNICATION: The word fornication is used in many ways throughout the

Bible and Scripture. It means in its broadest sense, any form of immoral (illegal) sexual activity. At the end of this chapter are many verses showing its sinful position in the eyes of your Creator.

Do not have any sexual contact of any kind with anyone if you are not married to that person. Being engaged is not married. Going steady isn't married. This means do not have any touching of genitals at all. Vaginal/penile intercourse needs to be absolutely avoided if you are not married. These areas should be covered and not touched by another unless you are married. If you are currently fornicating with someone, you can choose to repent and then make certain changes that will aid in walking in chastity, honoring your Creator, your body, and your unmarried health. Little changes, like not going to each other's homes or not having evening dates will help to remove opportunity. A good rule of thumb, is stay in public and daytime and modest touching, like holding hands, while you are not married.

PORNOGRAPHY and VOYEURISM both promote a type of fornication and adultery in the mind that can end in the actual act.

SODOMY: Sodomy has multiple acts that come under its heading. Two men together sexually is sodomy by definition. Semen is not food. Undigested semen passes through the intestinal wall causing a condition called autointoxication of the intestinal wall. Semen also contains immune suppression activity that passes through the absorbing intentional wall suppressing the immune system of the person being penetrated. (When semen is placed in the vagina of a monogamous couple, the natural immune suppression allows the sperm to reach the egg by temporarily lowering the woman's immune response. This is restricted to the vaginal area as it is the Creator's plan and the vagina is not designed for absorption like the intestines are). The stretching of the colon by thrusting and fisting damages the intestinal wall, allowing pathogens to freely pass over the intestinal wall. The vagina, however, stretches easily without damage and is not near blood vessels that can carry pathogens throughout the body.

Two women together sexually is lesbianism. This act is specifically mentioned as an unlawful, unnatural use of the body in Romans 1!

A man performing oral sex on a woman by placing his mouth on her genitals puts his digestive enzymes where they don't belong or may pass directly along harmful pathogens and harm her and IS ALSO SODOMY, MARRIED OR UNMARRIED, by definition. Her vaginal fluids which may contain pathogens will enter his digestive system and bloodstream through the mouth which is vascular and could harm him.

A man placing his penis into a woman's mouth is also sodomy, MARRIED OR UNMARRIED, by definition. It harms her immune system and damages the delicate tissue, and can throw semen and foreskin bacteria into her lungs and digestive system. Semen is not food and should not be placed in the digestive system.

A man placing his penis in a woman's anus is also sodomy, MARRIED OR UNMARRIED, by definition. Again, as in man with man sexual activity, this allows undigested semen to be absorbed by the colon causing autointoxication, and damages the tissues of the colon by the stretching and thrusting, allowing pathogens to cross the intestinal wall without first being made harmless by the upper digestive enzymes and probiotics. It also allows semen to enter the lower intestine and be absorbed undigested suppressing her entire immune system.

Even rear entry in a married, monogamous, heterosexual relationship can cause feces to be pushed into the vagina and urinary tract causing infections and some chronic conditions, like endometriosis.

There is speculation that a man performing anal sex, then vaginal sex with a woman may be the cause of endometriosis as it brings fecal matter into her vagina.

Mouths are for speaking, eating, and breathing. The anus is for elimination, exit only. These acts go against the natural use of the body and are forbidden for everyone, including married couples, as it is a deviant and destructive practice and called sodomy by very definition.

Placing SEX TOYS in the body is a type of sodomy and fantasy, conflicting with Creator intended intimacy that is to be between TWO people of the opposite sex that is supposed to exist during normal monogamous sexual activity.

Engaging sexually with animals also is a type of sodomy called BEASTIALITY. Again, this act conflicts with the Creator intended intimacy that is to be between 1 true and naturally born MAN and 1 true and naturally born WOMAN that is supposed to exist during normal monogamous sexual activity.

ADULTERY: When a person married to one person engages in sexual conductof any kind with someone who is not their husband or wife, it is called a blanket term adultery. If you have a husband or wife who is viewing pornography (lust for other people in the heart and voyeurism), pushing for deviant sexual acts, or is in an adulterous affair, you can become celibate and move to another room indefinitely for your own health and protection for as long as your spouse is engaging in deviant conduct as one possible solution. Messiah said that if a person even looks with lust in his heart, he has committed adultery in his heart already. The eyes and the thoughts break a trust and bond.

MASTERBATION: Self pleasure is an addictive behaviour, coming under a completely different sexual and mental category and can be classified as either adultery or fornication depending on its focus. In men, it harms the immune system because zinc, one of the pillars of the immune system, is lost in every ejaculation a man has. Continual masturbation depletes a man's immune system in time. Pathogens on the foreskin are transported up the penis in masturbation and can cause infections like prostate cancer and infections in the kidneys and bladder over time.

In women, beside the addictive behaviour that needs to come to a halt, it fosters isolation and possible labial, cervix, and vaginal infection.

Hebrews 13:4 KJV - Marriage [is] honourable in all, and the bed undefiled: but whoremongers and adulterers the Creator will judge.

When people honor their bodies with wholesome food, natural medicines, and wholesome treatment, they reap blessings and enjoy a hedge of protection from the Creator. When they choose to deviate from what the Scripture teaches, their lives are impacted negatively in many ways.

Romans 1:24-Wherefore the Creator also gave them up to uncleanness through the lusts of their own hearts, to dishonor their own bodies between themselves We are at this point in our worldwide society. It is the last days indeed.

FILTHY LANGUAGE-Avoid all sexualized slang and profanity, especially relating to marital intimacy. "Dirty talk" is profane, pornographic, degrading, crude, and sometimes violent.

Ephesians 5:4- Neither filthiness, nor foolish talking, nor jesting, which are not convenient: but rather giving of thanks.

Ephesians 4:29 - Let no corrupt communication proceed out of your mouth, but that which is good to the use of edifying, that it may minister grace unto the hearers.

Colossians 3:8-10 - But now ye also put off all these; anger, wrath, malice, blasphemy, filthy communication out of your mouth. Lie not one to another, seeing that ye have put off the old man with his deeds; 10 And have put on the new [man], which is renewed in knowledge after the image of him that created him:

Matthew 12:37- For by thy words thou shalt be justified, and by thy words thou shalt be condemned.

Colossians 4:6- Let your speech [be] alway with grace, seasoned with salt, that ye may know how ye ought to answer every man.

Matthew 15:10,11- And he called the multitude, and said unto them, Hear, and understand : 11 Not that which goeth into the mouth defileth a man; but that which cometh out of the mouth, this defileth a man.

2 Timothy - But shun profane [and] vain babblings: for they will increase unto more ungodliness.

Matthew 12:36- But I say unto you, That every idle word that men shall speak, they shall give account thereof in the day of judgment.

James 3:10- Out of the same mouth proceedeth blessing and cursing. My brethren, these things ought not so to be.

Philippians 4:8- Finally, brethren, whatsoever things are true, whatsoever things [are] honest, whatsoever things [are] just, whatsoever things [are] pure, whatsoever things [are] lovely, whatsoever things [are] of good report; if [there be] any virtue, and if [there be] any praise, think on these things.

Exodus 20- Thou shalt not take the name of the Creator your elohim in vain; for the Creator will not hold him guiltless that taketh his name in vain.

LUST VS. LOVE

All deviant sexual practices begin with lust. Lust and love are opposites. Lust is an evil destructive force that is ungodly and starts in the mind or carnal body. Lust is from Satan and encourages deviant sexual conduct which leads to death and destruction. Lust curses those involved and their children and grandchildren. It does not care about anyone or anything. When people give their minds over to lust they are putting Satan in the driver's seat. Lust leads to much destruction including adultery, fornication, rape, sodomy, beastiality, pedophilia, masturbation, and incest. Every destructive sexual behavior starts by allowing lust into your mind, giving one's mind over to Satan, who had come to kill, steal and destroy. And lust will do that to every area of your life. Giving one's mind over to lust is separation from your Creator. Lust is concerned ONLY about one's short term perceived need and blinds a person to future suffering.

Then, there is godly love and desire between a loving and monogamous husband and wife. When you are motivated by love you are motivated by doing what is pleasing to the Creator and obedience to His words and ways. It is willingness to sacrifice, to show restraint, and do what is best for the other person. This produces life and multigenerational blessings and health.

We are held responsible to make all thoughts obedient to our Creator. That means evil lustful thoughts must be rejected and not allowed to remain into your mind. "You can't stop a bird from flying over your head but you can stop it from building a nest in your hair" as the sayings goes. Many people pray as a conditioned response if a lustful thought enters their head and ask the Creator for forgiveness and help.

2 Corinthians 10:5 KJV- Casting down imaginations, and every high thing that exalteth itself against the knowledge of the Creator, and bringing into captivity every thought to the obedience of Messiah.

We must bring every thought and action under obedience to our Creator and Messiah.

HOW DO WE AVOID LUST?

To immunize your mind and heart against lust, learn what the Scripture teaches and guard your mind and heart. Do not expose yourself to lust.

Proverbs 4:23 Above all else, guard your heart, for everything you do flows from it.

Titus 2:12- Teaching us that, denying ungodliness and worldly lusts, we should live soberly, righteously, and godly, in this present world;

WHAT IS NORMAL, NATURAL SEX?

Normal sex is face to face, breast to breast, sexual contact between a married man and woman. Even in married terms, this form of sexual activity is SAFE and HEALTHY for BOTH partners.

WHAT DOES THE BIBLE SAY ABOUT THE NORMAL FREQUENCY OF SEX?

The Scripture says there is to be no sexual contact during a woman's menstrual period. If blood is present, there should be no sexual contact, well or ill. Blood vessels are open if blood is present so that semen or any pathogens present can possibly be forced into open vessels. For most women, this is 3 to 7 days of the month. Leviticus 18

The Scripture also commands that no sexual contact may take place 7 days after the last day blood is seen. This adds up to A TOTAL of 10 to 14 days of no sexual contact IN A ROW a month. This is protective for both the man and the woman. For the man, his reserves of zinc are replenished to keep his immune system high. For the woman, it gives her 10 to 14 nights a month to fully rest during her childbearing years when her life is the most stressful. The Creator is loving and merciful and these commands certainly show this for both the man and the woman. Leviticus 15

Beyond that, sexual contact can be anytime. Some abstain on the sabbath day and Scriptural feast sabbath days, also. Remembering other commands to wash the full body, all clothing, and bed clothing after each sexual contact is part of the commands concerning sexual activity.

IF I GET OR HAVE A SEXUALLY TRANSMITTED DISEASE, HOW DO I GET RID OF IT?

Sexually transmitted diseases can be viral, fungal, parasitic, or bacterial or a combination of any of these. The first thing you have to do is stop all sexual activity. If you are married, your husband or wife should be tested during this time, also. You both may have to stop sexual activity until both clear yourselves of the STD. This insures you do not re-infect each other. Following the regimens for parasites, then viruses and bacteria, then fungus will, in time, clear you of the infection.

We ARE free to behave however we want. We make our habits then our habits make us. Our prayers need to ask our Creator to help us make our greatest desire to do what He wants us to do and to put our selfish and fleshly desires to death. We CAN choose to reject ungodly desires and follow our Creator's desires for us. A wise person's greatest desire is to obey the Father in heaven.

However, the fruit of lust is trouble, sorrow, shame, disgrace, misery, death, and eternal damnation.

The fruit of the Holy Spirit is love, joy, peace, patience, kindness, goodness, faithfulness, gentleness, self-control and eternal life. Galatians 5

We will reap what we sow.

James 1:14-15 But each person is tempted when they are dragged away by their own evil desire and enticed. Then, after desire has conceived, it gives birth to sin; and sin, when it is full-grown, gives birth to death.

More verses that teach against deviant sexual practices-

1 Corinthians 6:13- Meats for the belly, and the belly for meats: but the Creator shall destroy both it and them. Now the body [is] not for fornication, but for the Creator; and the Creator for the body.

Galatians 5:16-24- [This] I say then, Walk in the Spirit, and ye shall not fulfil the lust of the flesh. 17 For the flesh lusteth against the Spirit, and the Spirit against the flesh: and these are contrary the one to the other: so that ye cannot do the things that ye would. 18 But if ye be led of the Spirit, ye are not under the law. 19 Now the works of the flesh are manifest, which are [these]; Adultery, fornication, uncleanness, lasciviousness, 20 Idolatry, witchcraft, hatred, variance, emulations, wrath, strife, seditions, heresies, 21 Envyings, murders, drunkenness, revellings, and such like: of the which I tell you before, as I have also told [you] in time past, that they which do such things shall not inherit the kingdom of the Creator. 22 But the fruit of the Spirit is love, joy, peace, longsuffering, gentleness, goodness, faith, 23 Meekness, temperance: against such there is no law. 24 And they that are Messiah's have crucified the flesh with the affections and lusts.

Revelation 21:8- But the fearful, and unbelieving, and the abominable, and murderers, and whoremongers, and sorcerers, and idolaters, and all liars, shall have their part in the lake which burneth with fire and brimstone: which is the second death.

Colossians 3:5-6 -Mortify therefore your members which are upon the earth; fornication, uncleanness, inordinate affection, evil concupiscence, and covetousness, which is idolatry: 6 For which things' sake the wrath of the Creator cometh on the children of disobedience:

I Timothy 1:8-11 - But we know that the law [is] good, if a man use it lawfully; 9 Knowing this, that the law is not made for a righteous man, but for the lawless and disobedient, for the ungodly and for sinners, for unholy and profane, for murderers of fathers and murderers of mothers, for manslayers, 10 For whoremongers, for them that defile themselves with mankind, for menstealers, for liars, for perjured persons, and if there be any other thing that is contrary to sound doctrine;

Romans 1:29 KJV- Being filled with all unrighteousness, fornication, wickedness, covetousness, maliciousness; full of envy, murder, debate, deceit, malignity; whisperers,

1 Corinthians 7:2 KJV- Nevertheless, [to avoid] fornication, let every man have his own wife, and let every woman have her own husband.

1 Corinthians 10:8 KJV- Neither let us commit fornication, as some of them committed, and fell in one day three and twenty thousand.

2 Corinthians 12:21 KJV- [And] lest, when I come again, my Creator will humble me among you, and [that] I shall bewail many which have sinned already, and have not repented of the uncleanness and fornication and lasciviousness which they have committed.

1 Thessalonians 4:3 KJV - For this is the will of the Creator, [even] your sanctification, that ye should abstain from fornication:

Jude 1:7 KJV - Even as Sodom and Gomorrah, and the cities about them in like manner, giving themselves over to fornication, and going after strange flesh, are set forth for an example, suffering the vengeance of eternal fire.

Revelation 2:14, 20-21 KJV - But I have a few things against thee, because thou hast there them that hold the doctrine of Balaam, who taught Balak to cast a stumblingblock before the children of Israel, to eat things sacrificed unto idols, and to commit fornication. ... 20 Notwithstanding I have a few things against thee, because thou sufferest that woman Jezebel, which calleth herself a prophetess, to teach and to seduce my servants to commit fornication, and to eat things sacrificed unto idols. 21 And I gave her space to repent of her fornication; and she repented not.

Revelation 9:21 KJV- Neither repented they of their murders, nor of their sorceries, nor of their fornication, nor of their thefts.

IS THERE A FORM OF BIRTH CONTROL THE CREATOR APPROVES ?

There are many forms of worldly birth control- abortion, birth control pills, IUD, condoms, creams, herbs that produce abortion, and more. Each of these hurt either mother, father, or baby, physically or chemically, or are not reliable 100% of the time. The book DOES THE BIRTH CONTROL PILL CAUSE ABORTION? explores and exposes some of these methods.

The only form of birth control that does not harm ANYONE is the mucus method. This method observes the 2 types of mucus a healthy woman produces and uses abstention for the approximately 100 hours each month a woman is fertile TO AVOID PREGNANCY. It is the natural way a woman can tell if she can get pregnant AT THAT MOMENT or not. IT IS FREE, AND HARMS NO ONE NOW OR FOR FUTURE ATTEMPTS AT GETTING PREGNANT. I believe it is the only truly safe and moral way to prevent or delay pregnancy and can be used monthly until menopause with no harm. I believe it is the heavenly Father's way of showing a woman if she is fertile and the only truly accurate way she can control her body as a nesting place for another baby in a time she chooses.

The book HOW TO AVOID OR ACHIEVE PREGNANCY NATURALLY explains this simple method.

HOW COMMANDED SCRIPTURAL CIRCUMCISM FOR MALES IS PART OF MEN'S AND WOMEN'S LONG TERM HEALTH

The Scripture commands all male babies to be circumcised on the 8th day after their birth. This practice is a covenantal sign of belonging to the Creator. It also is a health factor for both men and the women they marry. When the foreskin is removed, a hiding place for bacteria is removed. Men who are uncircumcised carry pathogens in the foreskin making infections more likely for them. Circumcised men have cleaner penises. Women who marry circumcised men have fewer cases of genital type cancer than women married to uncircumcised men.

This above chapter is a guest chapter co-authored with L. Francis, M.D.

CHAPTER 56

BASIC REGIMEN FOR TOTAL BODY CLEANSE IN 3 TO 6 WEEKS

This is a very intense total body cleanse that can be accomplished in as short a time as 3 weeks. It is like a boot camp for a complete health makeover. The person must be strong enough to handle all the supplements AT ONCE in this regimen. They must be able to digest and handle large quantities of liquids. I have seen some clients completely turn their health around VERY QUICKLY on this regimen, but it is not for the faint of heart as it is so concentrated. This kills parasites, viruses, bacteria, molds, fungus, pulls out toxins and chemical pollutants, restores digestive and bowel function and reestablishes beneficial bacteria in 3 weeks. Some choose to stay on this for up to 6 weeks to make sure all parasites are eliminated.

If you want to do this, make sure you can fully concentrate on it. It is best to set aside the time for it if you have to work and prepare everything for yourself. If you have help preparing the supplements and food, then working at a job is entirely possible.

Make sure you have EVERYTHING on hand before you start! And enough of all supplements for AT LEAST 3 weeks! Once you start, you do not want to stop until the healing is complete.

3 TO 6 WEEK TOTAL BODY CLEANSE

PRODUCT	WHEN ARISING	BREAKFAST	10:00 AM	LUNCH	3:00 PM	DINNER	BEFORE SLEEP	WHERE PURCHASED
PARATHUNDER	6							WWW.WHITESAGELANDING.COM OR PURE PLANET PARASITE CLENSE
NEEM CAPSULES	2			2		2		WWW.ALLABOUTNEEM.COM
HERBAL HEALER ACADEMY 500 PARTS PER MILLION COLLOIDAL SILVER		1/2 t.		1/2 t.		1/2 t.		WWW.HERBALHEALER.COM OR WWW.VITACOST.COM
KYOLIC ODORLESS GARLIC #101 OR #102		2		2		2		WAL-MART OR WWW.VITACOST.COM
COLONIX					½ SCOOP			WWW.DRNATURA.COM
BURIED TREASURE ACF		1 T.		1 T.		1 T.		WWW.VITACOST.COM
KLEARITEA						½ CUP		WWW.DRNATURA.COM
CO-ENZYME Q-10		3 TO 4 GRAMS						WWW.VITACOST.COM
GARDEN OF LIFE RAW ENZYMES		1 OR 2		1 OR 2		1 OR 2		WWW.VITACOST.COM
CARROT/PARSLEY JUICE		1 CUP		1 CUP				2 CUPS DAILY
RAW PROBIOTICS BY GARDEN OF LIFE VAGINAL CARE		2		2		2		WWW.VITACOST.COM
4 HERB TEA			1 CUP					WWW.HERBALHEALER.COM
ESTER, BUFFERED VITAMIN C		3,000 MGS		3,000 MGS		4,000 MGS		WWW.VITACOST.COM
LONGEVITY LOVE YOUR LIVER DETOX TEA					1 CUP			WWW.SHOP.LONGEVITYCORP.COM
LONGEVITY KIDNEY BLADDER DETOX TEA							1 cup	WWW.SHOP.LONGEVITYCORP.COM
OLIVE LEAF EXTRACT CAPSULES		1		1		1		WWW.VITACOST.COM
OREGANO OIL EXTRACT CAPSULES		1		1		1		WWW.VITACOST.COM
ORANGE COROMEGA		1 pak						WWW.VITAMINSHOPPE.COM

CHAPTER 57

HOW TO CURE YOURSELF OF ABOUT ANYTHING (NO KIDDING!)

If you do not know what CAUSES your health problem (and this can be true for many even doctor diagnosed conditions as there may be MULTIPLE infections where the doctor thinks there is ONLY one), there is a step by step plan you can use to systematically find out WHAT IS CAUSING your problem while you work on eliminating it. You will know when symptoms start going away during the step of the cleanse you are doing that that is the cause (or one of the causes).

To discover this yourself, do this step by step program. When you come to the actual thing that is causing at least part of your health problem, the symptoms will start going away as you work on that particular step. This is quite amazing and makes self healing easy and quite self-revelatory.

1. Cleanse kidneys with kidney cleansing herbal formula (Longevity Kidney Bladder Detox Tea). This is to prepare kidneys for all the waste it will soon filter.

2. If your problem is critical or chronic PERTAINING TO THE BOWEL OR INTESTINES ONLY, take one to four high enemas or colonics, spaced one or two days apart. Immediately, on the first day of the first colonic, start taking a comprehensive probiotic formula (Garden of Life Raw Probiotics for Women Vaginal Care- can be taken by men also- has 38 forms of probiotics)

3. Start eating only organic foods, focusing mainly on vegetables. Your diet should be at least 80% raw, fresh, and ripe as well as 100% organic.

4. Start drinking sufficient water or water plus herb teas (Longevity Love Your Liver Detox tea or Kidney Bladder Detox tea, 4 Herb Formula tea from Herbal Healer Academy, etc.) and freshly prepared organic juices. Water should be from a pure source (6 to 8 stage filtered, deep well, Penta-hydrate, Prima plant source bottled water, Zero filtered, etc.)

5. Remove all harmful chemicals from home, personal products, and food supply. This should already be done in the food area if you are eating only organically grown foods. A thorough clean up of your home and putting all chemicals in a non-roof sharing outside storage place will accomplish this. Replace all your personal care products with all natural ones with natural ingredients only (see list and sources in Chapters 49 and 53).

6. Start cooking in white Corning ware dishes, Fire King, Anchor Hocking, Pyrex, Glasbake, or any 100% glass or ceramic cookwear only.

7. Remove all mouth metal.

8. Remove silver colored fillings, posts, bridges, lined caps, and root canals containing metal. Replace with plastic or ceramic.

9. Start 3 week to 3 month herbal parasite cleanse (Parathunder, Pure Planet Parasite Cleanse and www.allaboutneem.com for neem). It can take about 3 weeks to 3 months to kill all the life stages of the over 200 types of parasites that can inhabit the human in some cases. Start #10 the same day.

10. Start virus and bacteria killing herbs (Buried Treasure ACF, Herbal Healer Academy 500 parts Per Million Colloidal Silver, Kyolic

Odorless Garlic #101 or #102, 10,000 mgs. daily ester, buffered Vitamin C) the same day as the parasite cleanse. Parasites release their stored and manufactured viruses and bacteria when dead. If you fail to do this, you may end up with multiple viral and bacterial infections.

11.   After 3 weeks, do a one day liver flush (see Chapter 26). All blood is filtered through the liver. As the clean-up continues, the liver and kidneys are working overtime, and need to be emptied of their stored refuse. Repeat every three weeks for the 3 months.

12.   After first 3 weeks or before, add mold, fungus, and heavy metal or chemical pollutant cleansing herbs and supplements (olive leaf extract capsules, oregano oil extract capsules, burdock tea, 1 bunch fresh cilantro for 3 weeks, Daily Detox tea (black box),Toxinout, etc.)

13.   If there are specific natural helps for your well known problem, use those specific substances to reverse your problem after the cleanses to fill in DEFICIENCIES.

Many clients notice at a very specific time when they start to feel better. It may be during the initial parasite cleanse, or while cleansing for molds, or when doing the first liver flush, etc. Each step is necessary in order to prepare for the next step.

Order of cleanses

Kidney cleanse (if you have been over exposed to heavy metals, solvents, or chemical pollutants; if not, proceed to next step) Kidney cleansing herb tea for 3 weeks at least 2 cups a day.

If your main health problem is in the bowel area, take 1 to 4 high enemas or colonics several days apart. Immediately start 15 or more form acidophilus/bifidus supplement. If not, proceed to the next step.
Herbal parasite cleanse and herbal anti-virals and anti-bacterials for 3 weeks to 3 months.

Take comprehensive 32 or more form probiotic, 10,000 mgs. Ester, buffered Vitamin C, and any other nutrients specific to your health challenge.

If your specific problem is digestive or intestinal, take a comprehensive digestive enzyme (Garden of Life Raw Enzymes, etc.) and a comprehensive probiotic formula (Garden of Life Raw Probiotics for Women Vaginal Care)

After 3 weeks, take one day liver flush.

At the beginning of 4th week, start kidney cleansing herb tea(Kidney/ Bladder formula at www.longevitycorp.com) at least two cups a day for three weeks if you have not already taken it.

At the beginning of the 5th week, start drinking 2 cups a day of Longevity(www.longevitycorp.com) Love Your Liver Detox tea. (This is not the same as the periodical "every 3 weeks" one day liver flush. These herbs restore the liver itself, strengthen its tissues, and also flush the contents gently over time.)

(After 6 weeks, 9 weeks, and 12 weeks, take a one day liver flush.)

Take mold and fungal cleanse for at least 3 weeks using 10,000 mgs ester, buffered Vitamin C, oregano oil extract capsules, olive leaf extract capsules, and 500 Parts Per Million Colloidal Silver fromHerbal Healer.com or Vitacost.com.

Take toxic metal and chemical cleanse for at least 3 weeks using Toxinout, burdock root tea or capsules, and one fresh bunch cilantro daily.

Every 6 months, take a one week herbal parasite cleanse.

OR

You can just go on the 3 Week Total Body Cleanse in Chapter 55!

CHAPTER 58

CLOTHING AND SHOES

Not many people stop to consider how clothing affects health. I am convinced that everything our Creator guides us to do through His commands is for our good, our protection, and our blessing in some way. His guidance on clothing issues falls into this caring category.

We are given guidelines in Scripture about clothing that few people think about...

Our Creator clothed men and women in robes of animals' skins. Since we know He stated later that we were not to touch the dead carcasses of Scripturally defined unclean animals, we can assume the animal skins were from Scripturally defined clean animals (cow, sheep, goat, deer, antelope, buffalo, etc). This shows, first of all, it is perfectly all right to kill animals, and it is all right to use animal skins for clothing. Animal skins give the body even temperatures throughout the system.

The robes or coats completely enveloped their bodies. The weight of the robes was suspended from their shoulders. This has been found to be the healthiest form of clothing as it causes no stress on the body. There are no major blood vessels crossing the shoulder. Suspending clothing from the shoulder does not hinder circulation in any way. It does not hinder circulation in any area of the body and allows free flow of air under the clothing.

YAHUAH told the priests to wear breeches under their clothing as a shield to other's eyes so their "nakedness" did not show when they ministered higher than the people in the tabernacle and temple. These breeches would be similar to our long underwear or long leg briefs of today. They were an UNDER garment, not seen on the outside as the robes they wore were LONGER than the breeches. Not once in Scripture does it mention women being given permission or commandment to wear these breeches under their robes or coats.

From a health standpoint, the clothing you wear should be very loose. It allows for circulation to proceed unhindered. Our custom of wearing tight EVERYTHING has contributed to digestive problems, breast problems, reproductive problems, back problems, and circulation problems which all can lead to degenerative problems as the body is starved of nutrition in some areas. The original coats or robes given to man by the Creator Himself showed the example of what clothing would be best for mankind—loose, long, covering, hanging down.

Tight pants women wear today can cause continual urinary tract infections. Underwire bras most certainly contribute to poor circulation in the breast area that can lead to cancer from poor circulation and lymph node congestion. Wide strap 100% cotton or 100% linen bras eliminate the solvent type fabrics and off gassing of foam inserts that pass into breast tissue. Wide straps spread out the weight of the breasts more evenly on the shoulder structure. Hiking the breast up too high by use of a bra can also put the breasts into an unnatural position and hinder circulation.

Long clothing covering most of the limbs prevents too much sunshine from shining directly on larges areas of skin ALL AT ONE TIME, RAISING THE BODY TEMPERATURE UNNECESSARILY. Loose clothing allows unhindered circulation and an even flow of air UNDER THE CLOTHING to allow even temperatures.

Our Creator said not to combine fibers in a clothing piece. (Leviticus 19:9; Deuteronomy 22:11) At that time it appears the only 2 things used for clothing were linen and wool. (The word "silk" is used in the Old Testament, but every time it is used, it is a different word. However, the New Testament uses the word for real silk from worms, and it is used in a negative way.) Each natural fiber has its own weight, wicking ability, and temperature controlling ability. Usually animal fibers are used in cold weather and vegetable fibers are used in warm weather. The modern combination of fibers (and combinations with solvent fibers) confuses the temperature setting mechanisms in your body that regulates keeping an even body temperature. (See Chapter 38 on single fiber fabrics and the sources of fibers).

Many of the fibers used today are products of the petro chemical industry. We have just started to understand all the damage of using these solvent type chemicals in and on our bodies. Natural fabrics of fibers or leathers are the healthiest types of fabrics in clothing, bags, loose belts, shoes, scarves, and boots.

LINEN IS THE BEST CHOICE FOR CLOTHING FABRIC AND BED LINENS.

Linen comes in several weights that can be used for any application from a light weight neck scarf to heavy upholstery or even rug material. Here are just a few of linen's superior and unique qualities...

There is evidence that using linen clothing assists in healing the body. The only plant fabric spoken of positively in the SCRIPTURES is linen. The priests were COMMANDED to wear linen in their service before the Creator in the tabernacle and temple.

It has the highest electronic cell energy (co-championed with wool) of any fabric material. Compared to the human cell energy of 70-90 units, its signature frequency is 5000 units of energy! All synthetic fabrics have ZERO cell energy. Cotton has between 40 and 100 units. Silk has 10 units. Rayon (made from plant cellulose) has 15 units. Any unit measure below 15 units is always associated with life threatening illness. Using linen keeps the energy around you very high and health giving!

Wearing linen and wool together as condemned by the Scriptures collapses the energy field from 5,000 units in each to ZERO WHEN COMBINED! In some cases, pain and weakness were measured when both were present. Interesting!

It is used in surgery inside the body because the human body can dissolve the linen cell once healing completes!

Linen fibers reflect light!

Linen protects against chemical exposure, noise, dust, solar gamma radiation, fungus, bacteria, bedsores, and decreases skin sores!

Linen absorbs water without feeling wet!

Linen has no known allergic factors and alleviates some other allergies!

Linen helps with inflammatory conditions, reduces fevers, helps neurological conditions as well as promotes good air exchange!

Linen does not conduct static electricity, has high air permeability, and heat conductivity (it feels cool in hot weather and warm in cold weather!!!)

Linen is moth resistant, resists dirt, rotting, and pilling. In other words it can last a long time in very good shape!

Linen can be boiled and heated without damage to the fabric!

Linen agriculture uses 5 times less pesticides and fertilizers than cotton in commercial non-organic growth!

Linen lasts 12 times longer than cotton and gets softer with age!

Linen does not shrink, and can be washed or dry cleaned!

SHOES

Shoes should be as flat as possible mimicking the natural steps of walking barefoot. Sandals with lots of open space are the best so that air and freedom of movement for the toes can be present. The biggest mistake people make in buying shoes is that they do not buy shoes WIDE enough for their feet. How freely, flat, and flexible you step every step affects circulation, posture, LONG TERM FOOT HEALTH AND LOWER LEG CIRCULATION, and duration of exercise.

Materials for shoes should be natural materials. It is very difficult to find 100% leather reasonably priced shoes now, but there are a few companies that are faithful to offer at least a few in their array of products. At the very least, only leather or vegetable fabric should actually touch your feet on the inside of the shoes. Many shoemakers offer that now.

Some good choices are Tom's Shoes, UGGS and other total sheepskin shoes, boots, and sandals, Naot, Terrasoles (if 100% leather), Italian Shoemakers,

Jambu, Birki's, Birkenstock, Mephisto, Robeez for kids, Jimmy Choo (if you can afford them!), Clark's, Patagonia, and Arche, are just a few that have SOME 100 % leather choices.

In the spring of 2010, a report came out that synthetic patent leather in many colors from China used in shoes, boots, purses, and belts contained over 10 times the amount of lead that our country allows in its manufacturing. Shoulder bags held next to the breast with some of these solvent and heavy metal pollutants in them can affect the lungs and breasts of the carriers. Use 100% leather and 100% cotton OR 100% linen (or other natural fibers) in purses, bags, shoes, loose belts, headbands, etc.

CHAPTER 59

FABRIC FIBER ORIGINS

The Scripture commands of not intertwining fibers for cloth for clothing, such as mixing linen and wool. Deuteronomy 22:11

The command of Scripture defines that the threads of a garment should not be of a mixed nature, but of purely one component. Some feel the assumption is that the clothing should be made only of naturally derived content, since wool, linen, and animal skins are mentioned in Scripture as materials for clothing, but this is not proven or solely commanded. Of course, for 98% of world history so far, only natural fibers have been used.

We are not told why not to mix fibers. It is known, however, that each natural fiber has its own temperature setting qualities, thickness, density, as well as its own wicking ability. We have also learned that each natural fiber has electronic cell energies measures in units. All synthetic fibers measure ZERO!

Many fabrics today in pre-made clothing have various mixtures of these fibers. Some fibers are from natural plants. Some fibers are from animal hair. Some fibers are from Scripturally unclean animal hair. Some are mixtures of natural and synthetic fibers. Some fibers are made like a plastic from vats of chemicals with no specific animal or plant origin. Some of the plastic types do come from a plant originally. Some fibers come from an earth material such as coal or sand. Some fibers are of undetermined origin or a mixture of many recycled fibers. Here is a list of various fibers available today and their origin.

NATURAL PLANT FIBERS

These fibers are used around the world for clothing and other uses. Quite often, these fibers are used for warmer weather clothing.

100% cotton

100% linen (flax)

100% flax (linen)

100% ramie

100% jute

100% kenaf

100% hemp

100% rattan

100% bamboo

100% vine

100% coconut fiber (coir)

100% raffia

100% pina (pineapple fiber)

100% sisal

100% fique

100% kapok

100% abaca (banana fiber)

100% seacell (from seaweed)

100% agave

These fibers are from plant cellulose-

Model (from beech tree cellulose)

Rayon (undetermined origin plant cellulose; could have several sources or types of trees in one batch)

Lyocell (undetermined origin plant cellulose; could have several sources in one batch)

NATURAL SCRIPTURALLY CLEAN (KOSHER) ANIMAL FIBERS

These fibers from kosher or Scripturally "clean" animals are used around the world for clothing and other uses. Quite often, these fibers are used for colder weather protection.

100% wool (sheep of various kinds)

100% mohair (Angora goat)

100% bison down (buffalo)

100% cashmere (Cashmere goat)

100% real pashmina (pashmina goat)

100% qiviut (from musk ox)

100% yak fur

100% merino (a specific sheep)

100% Cotswold (a specific sheep)

***********Llama, vicuna, guanaco, camel hair, and**********
alpaca are animal fibers of animals from the camel family, a Scripturally "unclean" animal family.

Catgut, sinew, avian fiber, feathers, or down can be from Scripturally "clean" or "unclean" animals.

Silk, horsehair, rabbit fur, mink, fox, beaver, wolf, leopard, sable, seal, chinchilla, zebra, civet, ermine, and many other normally named "fur animals" are also from Scripturally "unclean" animals.

TOTALLY SYNTHETIC FIBERS

These fibers are totally of synthetic origin. They start as a vat of chemicals and are spun into a thin plastic-like thread. There are no known animal or vegetable origins to these fibers. Each is made as a stand alone fiber. There are some fibers for clothing made with combinations of these fibers, however.

100% nylon

100% polyester

100% acrylic polyester

100% modacrylic

100% olefin

100% acrylic

100% carbon fiber

100% vinyon

100% saran

100% spandex (elastane?????)

100% ceramid

100% orlon or orlon acrylic

100% zylon

100% Kevlar

100% victran

100% dyneema (spectra)

100% PBI

!00% vinalon

100% nomex

100% urethane

100% polyurethane

100% twaron

NATURAL BASED SYNTHETIC FIBERS

These fibers are synthetic with a single, natural base.

Modal (synthetic from beech tree fiber)

However, these are from undetermined origin.

Rayon

Lyocell (Tencel)

LEATHERS

Most leathers are named from the animal they come from originally.

Cow leather

Sheep skin

Buffalo hide

Deer skin

Elk

Pig skin, alligator skin, snake skin, sting ray, kangaroo,
and ostrich hide are all leathers from Scripturally
*******"unclean" animals*******

NOTE! DO NOT USE GMO FIBERS- especially in tampons or diapers. Use organic forms of these personal items.

When my husband and I first got married he had some pigskin shoes. Right after he got the shoes, he got a very bad sore on his foot that would not heal even though the shoes fit him properly. He decided to get rid of the pigskin shoes because they were made of an unclean animal. In a few days, the sore healed!

Many fabric stores sell single fiber fabric to make clothing.

Fabric.com

Joann Fabric

Fashionfabric.com

Fashionfabriconline.com

Fabrics-store.com has hundreds of colors of linen in many different weights

And many more!

Many stores sell single fiber clothing, but you need to read the INDIVIDUAL labels carefully to see of what the clothing is made.

World Market

Cato

Chicos

Coldwater Creek

Gap

TJ Maxx, Marshall's, Ross

Oh My Gauze

Christopher and Banks

Eddie Bauer

LL Bean

Dune Gauze clothing

Land's End

Tommy Hilfiger

Steinmart

Hamricks

Bells of Florida

American Eagle

CHAPTER 60

DIGESTIVE, INTESTINAL, BOWEL, AND COLON PROBLEMS

Most digestive problems can be solved quite easily and quickly if a comprehensive digestive enzyme, comprehensive probiotics, and B complex vitamins are added very frequently to the diet. The first time the enzymes and probiotics are taken, a double or triple dose should be taken--4 to 6 capsules of each. Then take only 1 or 2 of each at every meal. If digestive symptoms are severe, take a water soluble B-100 complex tablet every hour on the hour every hour you are awake for 1 or 2 days. Sometimes this alone corrects intestinal problems within a day!!! Follow the Normal Bowel Function Restoration Diet (Chapter 41) for 3 to 10 days to rest the entire digestive system and soothe it.

If there is actual pain in the same place over the period of several days, you most likely have a parasite attached at that spot or the pain is caused by the waste products of the parasite. Take a thorough parasite cleanse and enteric coated peppermint tablets for a period of time.

If you know you have ulcers, use fresh cabbage juice while taking the parasite cleanse, along with goldenseal and myrrh capsules to kill the h. pylori present in ulcers.

Conventional meat, dairy, and eggs have residual amounts of many forms of antibiotics in them. These antibiotics kill the beneficial bacteria in your intestines. Therefore, if you use these or if you have used these in the past, you need to replenish your supply of beneficial bacteria daily. I suggest organic kefir probiotic drink to restore healing beneficial probiotic bacteria or Garden of Life Raw Probiotics for Women Vaginal Care.

CHAPTER 61

DIABETES AND ASTHMA

Many diabetics have lost their symptoms by using comprehensive digestive enzymes, taking a thorough parasite cleanse, eating more protein, and then adding a formula like Natrol Blood Sugar or KAL Blood Sugar Defense to fill in deficiencies after the cleanse.

Yamoa herb powder in honey is nearly a specific for true asthma. Over 85% of people with true asthma who took the yamoa powder in honey for a month lost all their symptoms. It kills the very specific parasite that is involved in true asthma. This is an African herb that is so valuable.

Some people with asthma-like symptoms need yamoa plus something else. This is because they may have the parasite that is killed by the yamoa AND OTHER PATHOGENS in their lungs. These people should do all the cleanses in order. Spraying the nasal passages and mouth while inhaling with Herbal Healer Academy or Vitacost 500 Parts Per Million Colloidal Silver has helped many more while taking the yamoa. Daily smelling or taking 2 drops of organic eucalyptus oil in a spoonful of honey helps soothe and open bronchial passages.

Olbas oil and eucalyptus oil placed by drop at the opening of the nostrils opens up breathing while taking the colloidal silver and yamoa so the vapors can shrink the swollen tissues and then the herb can enter the shrunken tissues via the circulatory system.

Michaels LNG formula, Ridgecrest Herbals Lung, and Nature's Secret Respiratory formula have herbs that clean the lungs. Both are very good formulas to use after other cleanses are done or after a lung infection to remove any left over mucus or debris. Liquid potassium iodide clears mucus from the lungs after an infection.

CHAPTER 62

ECZEMA AND PSORIASIS

Eczema and Psoriasis are two very difficult skin conditions to completely heal.

Eczema is a deficiency of certain fatty acids in the skin. I have seen many cases completely heal with the addition of 2 tablespoons organic, cold pressed corn oil for children and up to 4 tablespoons daily for adults while asking the client to completely eliminate commercial dairy products from their diet.

Psoriasis is more difficult than eczema to heal. Once the skin is broken and inflamed, there can be a combination of pathogens growing under the skin. Spraying Herbal Healer Academy 500 Parts Per Million Colloidal Silver on the skin or using a colloidal silver gel (CVS has this) or using Goldenseal/myrrh salve can help while taking the corn oil. Breaking open a probiotic capsule (non dairy} and wetting it with a few drops of water and rubbing it into the broken skin sometimes helps kill some of the pathogens. Some do very well with the B-100 Complex therapy 1 tablet or capsule every hour on the hour while awake. This helps take down inflammation and allergic reactions. Hanford's Balsam of Myrrh also kills many skin pathogens.

Sea salt baths and sea salt packs (wetting sea salt and making a poultice of it and leaving on the areas for 15 to 30 minutes) have helped many very difficult cases.

Neem soap from www.allaboutneem.com has been used to completely heal eczema and psoriasis. Lather thickly on problem areas. Leave on for 15 to 30 minutes 2 times a day. Rinse.

Always use a PH balanced soap and lotion on your skin.

CHAPTER 63

MISCELLANEOUS CURES

Hemorrhoids –grind several 600 mgs. rutin tablets. Mix with Vitamin E oil, or A and D ointment or Desitin. The paste must be very smooth. Apply to hemorrhoids several times a day. Take by mouth at least 600 mgs. rutin daily. This shrinks hemorrhoids sometimes in a day or two.

Sore throat - put one or two drops of eucalyptus oil in a spoonful of honey. Place in mouth and hold it there as long as possible, then swallow as slowly as possible. The aromatic oils will coat your throat while you are holding it in your mouth, and then the honey will coat your throat as it goes down. I have used this so many times to immediately stop a sore throat and so have my family and clients. Eucalyptus oil is antibacterial and somewhat antiviral. Honey can kill multiple pathogens. OR spray Herbal Healer Academy or Vitacost 500 Parts Per Million Colloidal Silver several times in the first hour.

Cuts or infected wounds - put honey on them to stop bleeding. Honey naturally coagulates and seals a cut. It has antibiotic and antifungal qualities. There is a medical doctor in our area who covers all diabetic sores with honey only!

Sinus infection - spray Herbal Healer Academy or Vitacost 500 Parts Per Million Colloidal Silver from a small spray bottle into nostrils, breathing in through nose very strongly as you spray. The mist coats your sinuses and kills over 650 pathogens on contact. It could be compared to being "Lysol for the throat"! This also kills sinus pain and throat pain very fast! OR inhale vapors from OLBAS oil and rub drops of the oil on sinuses, nose, neck and chest. Ridgecrest Herbals Sinus formula is very helpful, also.

Lung infections no one can diagnose - boil 2 quarts of water in a large soup pot; add several large spoonfuls of organic, raw honey. Get a towel and put it over your head and the pot. Breathe in the vapors of the honey and water. Do this twice a day until better. Russian scientists discovered, when given 17 impossible cases of various lung infections, that honey can cure nearly any type of infection of the lungs. All 17 cases got better. Some with 2 treatments all the way to some with 18 treatments, but all got better!

Shingles - As soon as blisters appear, make a tea of golden seal and myrrh (1 teaspoon of each in 2 cups of water). Bring to boil, boil one minute, let cool. When cool, take one clean cotton ball and soak the blisters and surrounding area with tea soaked cotton ball. Let air dry. Throw away cotton ball. Do this several times a day, and in a day or two the blisters and itching and pain will be gone! There is no residual pain with this treatment that can normally stay for months!

Poison ivy - take 2 to 4 activated charcoal capsules with a large glass of water. The charcoal will pull the poison ivy out of your skin INWARD! You can also put the charcoal right on the broken blisters and it will pull out the oil! I had poison ivy in my lungs two different times. This treatment saved me from a hospital visit each time. Do a second treatment in about 2 to 4 hours to complete the absorption!

Skin cancer - get a black salve like Cansema or other (must have bloodroot {sanguinaria} and cayenne in it). Put on once for 24 hours then pull off bandage. Use goldenseal/myrrh salve on it daily covered with a bandage until the cancer falls off! I have used this myselfand so have many of my clients!

Any type of infection of the mouth, throat, lungs or sinuses - Take Buried Treasure ACF a spoonful every hour. If you take this as soon as you feel a

278

battle going on in your body, you can stop an infection in 3 to 5 hours! So many of my clients have used this and reported back to me I wonder if the Buried Treasure Company made their formula from my proven single ingredients combination before this product ever came out! Or Spray Herbal Healer Academy or Vitacost 500 Parts Per Million Colloidal silver on any infected part.

TB- Drink yerba santa tea. It kills it in a few days!

Upper body chest tumors and breast tumors - drink sanicle tea along with a good cancer regimen. This tea has been used for years to shrink upper body tumors very effectively!

Tumors- take Barley Max 2 or 3 times a day- I have seen tumors shrink in 3 days using this with Essiac.

Clean mucus out of the lungs after a lung infection – drink vervain and yerba santa tea-3 cups a day. OR use potassium iodine, 10 drops per ½ cup of water. A medical doctor told me of this natural remedy and it works very fast to dry up lung mucus!

Apple cider vinegar - whole books have been written on ACV, but the most beneficial use I feel is that when your stomach is upset or you think you may have a stomach bacteria or virus. Drink 2 or 3 tablespoons in a cup of water. It kills bacteria and viruses on contact. The nausea will stop in a few minutes and all the symptoms will fade.

Honey - Whole books have also been written on the use of honey as medicine, but one of the best is if you have acid reflux. Taking a couple of spoonfuls of honey before bed stops acid reflux!

Hair loss and hair regrowth – many people start losing hair during times of great stress. Mix equal parts of organic smooth peanut butter and Plantation blackstrap molasses. Eat 1 to 3 tablespoons of the mixture daily. Most see tiny hairs growing within the first week! This combination contains every mineral and nutrient needed to regrow hair. I have had so many people use this successfully!

If you want to kill off a COLD or INFECTION RIGHT WHEN IT STARTS—
As soon as you feel a battle going on inside your body, start taking a
tablespoonful of Buried Treasure ACF and teaspoonful of Herbal Healer Academy or Vitacost 500 Parts Per Million Colloidal Silver every hour on the hour for 3 to 5 hours. This is one of my personal classic remedies that ALWAYS WORKS no matter what the infecting pathogen. If you kill the growth of the pathogens before they multiply exponentially, you can get better in a few hours! This one remedy alone has saved my clients days of sickness and hours of misery and thousands of dollars in doctor visits and drug bills! A few drops of lemon grass oil, lemon oil, pine needle oil, or eucalyptus oil in a spoonful of honey or empty veggie capsules or a few capsules of goldenseal are also very effective.

CHAPTER 64

PARASITE, VIRUS, BACTERIA, MOLD, AND FUNGUS KILLERS; HERBS FOR REMOVING HEAVY METAL AND POLLUTANT CHEMICAL

These things kill PARASITES safely---

Green black walnut hulls, neem, wormwood, cloves, garlic, onions, pumpkin seeds, fennel seeds, pomegranate juice, carrot juice, elderberry, bilberry, the herbal combination in Buried Treasure ACF, Herbal Healer Academy or Vitacost 500 Parts Per Million Colloidal Silver, clove oil, fennel oil, Hanford's Balsam of Myrrh (topical only!), myrrh, golden seal, parsley, Miror Core Miror EPF, and neem.

These things kill VIRUSES safely---

Ester, buffered Vitamin C, myrrh, goldenseal, elderberry, aloe vera, bilberry, pine needle oil capsules, garlic, neem, lemon juice, orange juice, tangerine juice, grapefruit juice, echinacea, eucalyptus, etrog (wild lemon of Israel), Young Living Thieves Essential oil blend, Buried Treasure ACF, Herbal Healer Academy or Vitacost 500 Parts Per Million Colloidal Silver, apple cider vinegar, and Hanford's Balsam of Myrrh (topical only!), lemon oil, tangerine oil, grapefruit oil, orange oil, bergamot oil, frankincense oil, myrrh oil

These things kill BACTERIA safely---

Honey, Buried Treasure ACF, eucalyptus, garlic, peppermint, myrrh, goldenseal, lemon, etrog (wild lemon of Israel), apple cider vinegar, neem, Buried Treasure ACF, Herbal Healer Academy or Vitacost 500 Parts Per Million Colloidal Silver, Young Living Thieves essential Oil Blend, and Hanford's Balsam of Myrrh (topical only!), lemon oil, frankincense oil, myrrh oil

These things kill MOLDS safely ---

Vitamin C spray, ester, buffered Vitamin C (10,000 mgs. daily) taken internally, acerola, lemon, etrog of Israel, lemon oil, Young Living Thieves oil and Thieves products, and neem.

These things kill FUNGI safely---

Oregano oil extract, olive leaf extract, myrrh, garlic, lemon, lemon oil, orange oil, goldenseal, Herbal Healer Academy or Vitacost 500 Parts Per Million Colloidal Silver, Buried Treasure ACF, neem, frankincense oil, Hanford's Balsam of Myrrh (topical only!)

These things remove HEAVY METALS and CHEMICAL POLLUTANTS safely---

Daily Detox tea (black box), Toxinout, fresh cilantro daily for 3 weeks, burdock tea, 4 Herb Formula tea and capsules by Herbal Healer Academy, Flor-Essence, Essiac tea or capsules, garlic, chlorella, and milk thistle.

CHAPTER 65

THE MOST LOVING THING I HAVE EVER SEEN

Anna, 21, had one spot of cancer on the back of her tongue.

She worked for her Dad in a carpet and upholstery cleaning business using many strong solvents. The church she belonged to believed in prayer and divine healing in specific cases. She was prayed for by her grandfather, a missionary to many destinations in the Far East. It appears that the cancer was gone, but the tumor remained, so her parents wanted her to get radiation treatments for the tumor. She received treatments from a brand new machine with a newly trained technician. Apparently, either the technician was not trained well or the machine was defective or not calibrated correctly, and Anna received terrible radiation burns on her tongue, cheeks, gums, and throat.

Just by chance (of the Heavenly Father), a friend of the ministry who was a radiation treatment nurse came to the church to visit. He said the symptoms she was suffering were typical of radiation burns. He said the skin would swell up, slush off, and new pink skin would be underneath. He said it could be a long time before the process would be complete. The time mentioned was MONTHS!

By the time I was called to see if I knew anything that could help her, her face was so swollen she looked like something from a horror movie. Her chin was about 3 inches longer than it was supposed to be with a large drainage hole in it. Her gums and tongue were so swollen that she could not swallow or even close her mouth, so a stomach tube and neck placed breathing tube were necessary. Pieces of flesh were breaking off in her mouth daily.

The church group had bought a home near the church to be used just for Anna. They completely remodeled the home and furnished it with cheerful furnishings. There were beautiful hangings and pictures with Scripture verses scattered throughout the home. There was a huge plate glass front window in the living room area where they placed Anna's hospital bed. There were beautiful flowering bushes, a large yard, and birdfeeders placed outside the window.

Two angel registered nurses worked 12 hour shifts daily, taking care of Anna's every need. They wiped the saliva that constantly dripped from her mouth EVERY FEW MINUTES and suctioned the saliva and slushed off flesh that fell back in her throat. Church members came in with cooked food for her parents who stayed by her bed and had rooms to sleep in when necessary. Members cleaned the home as needed. Many came to visit and to pray and to encourage Anna and her helpers. Sometimes someone would break out into spontaneous song and all in the home would join in. Some would at times break out into spontaneous encouragement by speaking Scripture verses or personal encouragement to Anna. There were tapes of Scripture based music available for Anna to hear whenever she desired.

All involved were willing to ANYTHING it would take to help Anna get well. Love flowed in the home. It was so beautiful. I wished every church could have seen the example of how sick people are to be taken care of in the church. What they had provided there was an actualization of the many thoughts I had had in the past of what I envisioned health care in the church should be.

The grandfather, the grandmother, and some of Anna's friends and relatives knew I did home natural care and counseling and asked me to come to see what I could do for her. They told me she had had cancer and was recovering. I was a little puzzled at first when I saw her as it did not look as if the swelling or

284

raw areas were cancer I had seen before. Then they told me of the radiation burn possibility.

I designed a program for her to treat POSSIBLE leftover cancer, swelling, toxin removal, and tissue repair. She weighed 86 pounds and had not had a bowel movement in many WEEKS when I arrived. Within 5 days, after feeding her through a stomach tube, she had gained 5 pounds with several bowel movements occurring. The swelling was going down, and there was an acceleration of the dead tissue slushing off.

The two nurses, Helen and Stella, who were helping her, were so eager to learn a natural way of treating her. They had absolutely no experience in doing natural and herbal treatments and were attentive students, learning all they could, asking pertinent questions, willing to follow any regimen, no matter how tedious, to get Anna well again. I felt very humbled to have such excellent help consistently following the regimen I hoped would bring Anna back to her young, vivacious, beautiful self. I had had similar experiences with families pulling together, making schedules, preparing the elements for the regimens for a patient after I had taught them what to do, making sacrifices, losing sleep while treating patients when they had to go to work the next day. But it was a personal lofty and seemingly impossible dream of mine to see registered nurses with all their experience and training and their knowledge of sanitary procedure in a specifically controlled beautiful environment help someone in desperate condition progress using only all natural things.

Anna progressed. Everyone around her knew she had made progress. After 5 days, I had to leave because my own son got sick and was in the hospital. I knew everything was under control and in good hands when I left Anna. Everyone there knew they could call me at any time if they had questions or if problems needed to be solved. I also knew it could be months before Anna was really well. I wondered if the nurses could sustain the energy needed to care for Anna 12 hours a day 7 days a week with no rest for several months. I hoped the nurses did not burn out.

That was the beautiful part..now the not so beautiful part...

One morning about a week later I woke up and knew something was wrong. I saw as a vision Anna's swelling going down in the back of her throat and some of the back tongue material slushing off and passing down her now opened throat into her lungs. After the vision ended, I called the nurse Helen and told her she needed to suction the back of Anna's throat so that none of the slushing dead material went down into her lungs as the swelling went down and her throat opened up. She told me she was a little reluctant to do that as she was afraid she might disturb some of the material by doing this. I told her she had to do this or Anna might end up with pneumonia.

The very next day Anna was admitted to the hospital with pneumonia because material had gone into her lungs!!! She took antibiotics which took care of the pneumonia in a few days. From that day forward, the doctor who had ordered the radiation (and knew Anna could have sued him and the hospital for their very lives because of the defective radiation treatment) told the parents Anna could never get better, so THEY could administer morphine from an IV pump whenever THEY desired to keep their daughter from pain. (She was in no pain at the time!) Anna, who could not speak, wrote a note to her grandmother, present in the room, stating she knew they were trying to kill her and get this over with.

The cause of death was not cancer or radiation poisoning. Anna died from morphine poisoning within a few days.

Anna had only on small spot of cancer on the back of her tongue...

The most loving thing I had seen was the care and provision the church had made for her to recover, which she would have done if natural treatment had been followed after the pneumonia was under control. The pastor, her grandfather, wrote me a beautiful letter after all of this happened telling me he knew she WAS GETTING and COULD have gotten COMPLETELY better if the treatment had been followed and thanked me for all my help to them.

CHAPTER 66

THE HOME NATURAL MEDICINE CHEST

Keep these things in your home to treat many things naturally. I keep these things in my home at all times to have on hand some very simple, yet comprehensive remedies to address health problems as soon as they appear. Doing this cuts down the actual time being sick. Remember, most pathogens grow exponentially. If you stop their growth while the numbers are small, you can recover much more quickly and use fewer of your reserves stored to fight future infections!

In cabinet or cupboard -
Apple cider vinegar
Honey
Baking soda
Aloe vera gel (pure)
Herbal Healer Academy or Vitacost 500 PPM Colloidal Silver ina spray bottle
Neem capsules
Oregano oil extract capsules
Olive leaf extract capsules
Goldenseal/myrrh capsules
Lugol's solution
Activated charcoal powder in caps
Ammonia
Young Living Thieves, Eucalytus, Lemon, Orange, Cinnamon, Frankincense, Myrrh, Sacred Mountain, Pine Needle, Lemongrass, Blend oils
Olbas oil
Olbas cream
Penn Herb goldenseal/myrrh capsules

Burt's Bees lip balm in round tin

Hanford's Balsam of Myrrh liquid tincture

Peppermint tea bags

Swiss Kriss tea

Fresh garlic

Refrigerated –

Buried Treasure ACF

Garden of Life Raw Probiotics for Women Vaginal Care- 38 forms

Buried Treasure Prevention

Elderberry syrup

Lemon juice

Garlic oil

Raw Enzymes by Garden of Life

CHAPTER 67

RELIABLE ORGANIC COMPANIES

There are so many reliable and time proven organic companies right now from whom you can buy canned foods, dried foods, frozen foods, and skin care products (remember, everything you put on your skin can end up in your bloodstream, just like a food!)

What to Look For In Foods and Products

When looking for REAL FOOD, it should be organically grown and with no added chemicals in the food or product. What you buy to go in or on your body should be an organic, whole food product. If it is encapsulated it should be with vegetarian or kosher or bovine capsules, and/or standardized for the herbal active ingredient.

There are so many companies that produce excellent products now. I always look for the best product for the purpose that needs to be accomplished. The products I choose will almost always have what I need and want in them plus some more ingredients to make them all the more comprehensive. This is just a partial listing. There are many more companies, and new companies and products are being introduced all the time!

The Besorah Seed www.allaboutneem.com

Paul Nison's www.RawLife.com

Garden of Life

Aloe 1

Arrowhead Mills

Walnut Acres

Muir Glen

Cascadian Farms

Earthbound Farms

Eden Foods

Small Planet Foods

Purely Organic

VerdeGrass

Annie's Natural

Respect Organics

The Raw Food World

Organic Kingdom

Sun Organic Farm

Diamond Organics

Terressentials Personal Care Products

Michael's

Rainbow Light

Source Naturals

Dr. Amen's

Nutiva

Young Living Essential Oils

Baker Seed Company

Reservage

www.nuts.com under organic

www.vitacost.com

NEVER USE ANY SKIN PRODUCT THAT IS BLUE! Blue coloring means there is cobalt in it in very high concentrations! Excessive cobalt (cumulative through frequent use) is indicated as one causative factor in many modern diseases! Watch the blue popsicles, too!

Remember, any chemical in personal care products that has the "propyl" prefix is a possible associative and causative factor for cancer!

CHAPTER 68

SOURCES FOR ESSENTIAL SUPPLEMENTS

All of these supplements are either with kosher capsules, made exclusively with bovine gelatin (beef) capsules, or are a total vegetarian formula. This is not a complete list. There are new and better products being formulated all the time. There are MANY, MANY more than these. Remember to always check your labels as ingredients and formulas change frequently in products

Comprehensive Digestive Enzymes---

Vibra-gest by Nature's Plus-11 enzymes, 3 form acidophilus--first choice tie

Raw Enzymes by Garden of Life – 22 enzymes—first choice tie

Total Enzyme by MicroTech-14 enzymes

Multi-Enzyme by Natural Factors-13 enzymes

13 Powerful Digestive Enzymes by Nature's Secret - 13 enzymes

UltraZyme by Nature's Plus-12 enzymes, 3 form acidophilus

Acti-Zyme by Nature's Plus-12 enzymes, 1 form acidophilus

Enzymedica Digest Gold-12 enzymes, 1 form acidophilus

Peaceful Digestion by Veg Life-11 enzymes

Super Enzymes by NOW-10 enzymes

Mega-Zyme by Enzymatic Therapy-10 enzymes

There are many more enzyme/probiotic formulas. I have chosen to only list those with 10 enzymes or more in the above list. If you are going to spend your money on enzymes, get a formula with the most individual enzymes.

Parasite Cleansing---

HERB

(This herb combination must contain at least green black walnut hulls, wormwood, and cloves)

Parathunder by White Sage Landing– first choice—

Pure Planet parasite cleanse

Wormwood combo by Eclectic Institute (Dr. Hulda Clark formula)

Clear by Assurance Corp.

Vermex by Crystal Star

Wormwood Combo by Kroeger Herb

Paraherbs by Michael's

Parex Intensive Care by Metagenics

Paragone by Renew Life

Parathunder

Dr. Floras

Parakids by Renew Life (for children)

Cedar Bear Children's Parasite Cleanse (for children)

Humaworm

COMPLETE PACKAGE

Paragone by Renew Life

Natural Medicine Associates-complete parasite cleanse

(liquid, fiber powder, herb capsules)

1-800-388-7012

Calcium/Magnesium combinations---

This combination should contain calcium (preferably 3 to 6 forms of calcium), magnesium, Vitamin D, and boron, at least)

Bluebonnet Nutrition Osteo-Bone formula-the best

Source Naturals Ultra Bone Balance tabs-the best

Buried Treasure Calcium Plus liquid – very good

Country Life Calcium/Magnesium 1000 mgs./500 mgs. tabs

Country Life Calcium/Magnesium/Zinc tabs

Nature's Plus Nutrical tabs

New Chapter Cal/Mag

Rainbow Light Food-based Calcium tabs

Lowe's Foods Cal/Mag with Boron and Vit. D - complete

Swanson Vitamins Liquid Cal/Mag/Vit. D/Boron

Green Foods---

Barley Max – first choice for cancer

Green Vibrance –first choice for rebuilding

Organifi Green

Perfect Food - Garden of Life

Pines Wheat Grass or Green Barley

Green Magma by Japan Natural Foods

Kyo-Green by Wakunga

Pro-Greens by Nutricology

Barley Grass by Solar Green

Daily Blue Green Algae

Barley Juice Powder by Nature's Sunshine

Mighty Greens

Barlean's-no sugar

Barley Green by AIM
Reservage

Fiber Products---

This should contain ground flaxseed

Colonix by Dr. Natura—first choice
Wal-Mart Equate
Fiber Smart by Renew Life (powder only)
Natural Medicine Associates fiber

Garlic---

Kyolic Odorless Garlic (vegetarian formula) # 100

Chlorophyll liquid---

Bernard Jensen's Mint Flavored Chlorophyll Liquid

Cancer Herb Formula---

This should contain at least burdock root, sheep sorrel, slippery elm, and turkey rhubarb

4 Herb Formula - Herbal Healer Academy
Trout Lake Farm Camas Prairie Tea
Essiac
Flora Flor-Essence
Can-ssiac by Crystal Star

Golden Seal/ Myrrh caps---

Penn Herb

Neem products---

www.allaboutneem.com

Colloidal and Ionic Silver
This should contain very high PPM and very small microns of silver

Herbal Healer Academy 500 PPM colloidal silver—first choice
www.vitacost.com -500 PPM colloidal silver

General Immunity –

Buried Treasure ACF—first choice
Any Source Naturals Wellness formula

Acidophilus choices---

This should contain many forms of probiotics. The more, the better.

Raw Probiotics for Women by Garden of Life, Vaginal Care –38 strains of
acidophilus and bifidus - first choice
LB -17 -17 strains
Flora Source -16 strains
Nutraceutical Sciences Institute Probiotic 15-35 – 15 strains
Primal Defense by Garden of Life-14 strains

Mega Foods Mega Flora - 14 strains, refrigerated

New Chapter Probiotics With A Purpose-Sensitive Colon Support-10 strains

New Chapter Probiotics With A Purpose- Cold and Flu –10 strains, refrigerated

New Chapter All Flora - 9 strains

Nature's Life Lactobacillus Probiotic Liquid (blueberry)-7 strain acidophilus, refrigerated, fructose only

(strawberry-apple) 1 strain acidophilus, honey only

Solaray Multi-dophilus Powder-3 strains acidophilus, refrigerated

Renew Life Flora Bear-3 strains, refrigerated

Country Life Maxi Baby-dophilus - 6 strains

Solgar Acidophilus

Solgar Acidophilus Plus

AND

Ridgewood Hill Farm plain goat yogurt-no sugar- 4 form acidophilus, refrigerated

AIDS/HIV Aftercare---

Natrol My Defense

Heavy Metal Cleanse---

Renew Life Heavy Metal Cleanse and Daily Detox

Crystal Star Heavy Metal Cleanse

Daily Detox Tea-black box

Toxinout by Dr. Natura

Lung Cleanse---

Michaels LNG formula

Ridgecrest Herbals ClearLung

Nature's Plus Ageloss Lung

Kidney Detox---

Longevity Kidney and Bladder Detox tea

Liver Detox---

Longevity Love Your Liver Detox tea

Kid's Multiples---

These have no artificial colors or flavors.

Country Life Tall Tree

KAL Dinosaur Eggs

Nature's Plus Animal Parade

Natural Factors Big Friend

Twin Labs Animal Friends

Yummy Bears (Gelatin Free Type Only)

Companies are always changing their formulas. Check your labels and capsule contents.

New companies are always forming with new great products. Look for organic, vegan, and kosher for the contents and veggie, vegetable, bovine, or kosher for the capsules.

CHAPTER 69

IF YOU ARE THE CAREGIVER

I HAVE WORKED WITH MANY LOVING FAMILIES AND FRIENDS OF VERY SICK PEOPLE WHO HAVE WORKED HARMONIOUSLY TOGETHER TO HELP THE ILL ONE GET WELL. These people just wanted to know and do what had to be done to bring their loved one back to good health. They worked tirelessly and with great cooperation, enthusiasm, and willingness to learn all they could in the natural treatment area to help their loved one. They worked cheerfully and hopefully with each other, buying organic foods, preparing foods, ordering supplements, making juices and teas, portioning out mealtime supplements, keeping a regular schedule, and sometimes bathing and feeding the client until the client was strong enough to help himself. They spread the load of helping the client amongst themselves, so not just one person would have the burden of helping, making schedules of times to come to care for the client. In most cases, I taught one or more of the group how to do all that was needed in these areas, and then that one taught the others who came to help in the clients home.

If you are planning on helping someone in this way, there are several things you must know-

The whole area of living must be cleaned and kept clean.

The personal hygiene of EVERY SINGLE PERSON entering the home must be considered. Everyone should wash hands frequently.

Anyone touching the food, juices, teas, or supplements must wash hands frequently and make sure all preparation utensils are well washed.

The noise level in the home should be dictated by the client, not the helpers. Healing takes place restfully in quiet conditions. Most clients sleep a lot during recovery and need a quiet atmosphere to sleep and heal.

Once the plan of action is determined by the patient, there should be no more discussion or discouragements to the patient. He or she has decided what THEY want to do with their health. As the saying goes, "lead, follow, or get out of the way"!

Consistency and persistence are keys in healing naturally. Most healing goes on when the client is asleep after taking the healing agents. It takes days to heal completely from a ravaging and devastating disease, but healing comes relatively quickly if consistent treatment is given. I have seen it over and over again. It works if good and right treatment is repeated until the total healing appears.

CHAPTER 70

SEND A MESSAGE, GET READY TO STAND, AND LEAVE A LEGACY

I want to encourage you. There are many changes you must make to achieve really good health. The thing that is so sad is that these changes would not be necessary if we had not changed to unhealthy choices many years ago. The truth, however, remains; we cannot fully get well without reversing these practices that have given us poor health.

You have to be determined and set your course once you decide to live on a higher plane for your health's sake and your children's health sake, but the rewards are great if you do. I had 8 children. My children ate all natural foods all the time they were growing up. They had very happy dispositions, were gentle and kind, hardly EVER got sick, received no immunizations and yet got none of the regularly feared children's early childhood diseases (except chicken pox! They came down with them one by one about every half hour after a visit from relatives who had just been exposed to the virus. They had symptoms for about a day each and did have a few sores, but it passed very quickly and healed very quickly.)

There is truth in every aspect of life. You have the choice to reject it or embrace it and its favorable destiny. All you do today affects your children and grandchildren in the future! How beautiful and noble it is to make a change for the better! How brave and forward thinking it is to make decisions whose effects reach far into the future!

CHAPTER 71

ORGANIC NOW!

Organic Now! is an organization and a movement to encourage everyone to buy only and consume only organically grown foods and products. It was established to encourage our lawmakers to enact laws that would prohibit anything but organically grown products to be commercially produced in, sold in , and imported to the USA and exported to the world.

If this movement grows, the society would see fewer birth defects, fewer cases of modern diseases, a cleaner water supply, cleaner air, fewer cases of cancer and other degenerative diseases, and more jobs in the original occupation, organic gardening.

Join me in insisting on our government promote only the advancement of organic commercial agriculture for the PROTECTION OF THE PEOPLE LIVING NOW AND FOR FUTURE GENERATIONS! It is our responsibility to protect our children and grandchildren in this matter!

CHAPTER 72

SOME OF MY OBSERVATIONS OVER 37 YEARS AS AN HERBALIST

The people I have known who have had the most severe and frequent doctor defined asthma attacks have all had cats in their homes and usually let them run anywhere in their homes the cats desired including the kitchen counters and sleeping pillows.

Almost every person I have known who has had leukemia or died from leukemia had previously eaten eggs very frequently, usually farm eggs or eggs from non-Rous vaccinated chickens and/or had cats in their homes.

Nearly everyone I have known who ate fins and scales fish exclusively for animal protein remained at a healthy weight.

Most of the complete lacto ovo vegetarians I have known who included sugar in their diets had weight problems, heart problems, and/or eye problems.

Several people I have known who ate commercial beef exclusively (no other types of meat) for animal protein had cow like proportions to their bodies.

Many people I have known whose chief source of animal protein was pork (bacon, ham, sausage, luncheon meat, etc.) had pig like looks. This is not a joke. I have asked several of my natural practitioner friends if they had ever observed that and they said yes!

Most people I know who eat a lot of commercial dairy products have been overweight or constantly struggled with their weight.

Many women I have known with naturally very soft, feminine characteristics who ate a lot of commercial dairy products came down with cancer sometime during their lives.

CHAPTER 73

IF I WERE PRESIDENT, IF I WERE PRESIDENT

There are some things that need to be fixed in this country that very few are willing to risk their money and lifestyles on to be a part of real progress. Nevertheless, these things need to be addressed for the protection and good welfare and healthy future of the people of this country. Consider these suggestions and solutions...

Organic agriculture only should be instituted.

Since it is known degenerative disease is caused mostly by half foods being sold as real food, any food that does not contain whole foods should be taxed as a luxury item OR COMPLETELY OUTLAWED.

For instance, for every gram of sugar over 2 grams that a cereal contains per serving, that cereal should be taxed a percent. If a cereal has 11 grams of sugar per serving then there should be an additional 9% tax on it. And this tax should go into Medicare and Medicaid to help pay for future medical care. This would encourage cereal makers to make good tasting, low sugar cereals and tax those who continually use these cereals to eventually pay for THEIR OWN MEDICAL BILLS WHICH SHALL SURELY COME IF THEY CONTINUE TO EAT THESE HIGH SUGAR CEREALS. The same principle could be applied to grams of saturated fats per serving, milligrams of sodium, grams of sugars in baked goods and drinks, grams of saturated fats, percentage of white flour and white rice in prepared foods, etc. It would force users of these products to "pre-pay" their own medical bills which will surely come in the future!!! And those who do not purchase these products would not be affected by this added expense in any way.

The agriculture of tobacco should be outlawed. There is not one good thing that comes out of its production. Programs such as are now being offered in North Carolina and other states can retrain farmers and refit their farms to be able to grow other crops and purchase the equipment to grow alternative crops.

Interest free loans should be available for those farmers willing to go into organic farming, herbal agriculture, start vegan restaurants, and commercial goat farming and other better farming practices.

The production of any beverage over the alcohol content of 3% should be totally outlawed. Again, there is not one good thing that comes out of the consumption of alcoholic beverages. Roads would be safer, children of drinkers would have more food and clothing, physical abuse would decrease, SOME TEENAGERS WOULD LIVE LONGER, there would be fewer alcohol related health problems for the health care system to deal with, and the general health of the former drinker would increase.

The use of any non-natural fertilizer, pesticide, or herbicide should be outlawed. Any food sold should be whole and organic. Companies such as The Necessary Company and Gardens Alive have shown commercial agriculture can flourish without damaging the environment or poisoning the food or water supply.

Full tax credits should be given to anyone, up to the whole of their one year's tax, who installs any wind, solar, geo-thermal, instantaneous water heaters, or any other energy saving devices in their homes or businesses.

There should be abundant research in the area of whole herbal medicine for the cure for diseases.

CHAPTER 74

LEGACY (I HOPE!)

If I could die and be remembered for THESE things, I hope it would be "she lived in faith, love, and obedience to Scriptures AND URGED OTHERS TO TASTE AND SEE THAT THE CREATOR IS GOOD" and "she told the world to get rid of their parasites and showed them how" and "she told the world of the deadly effects of living in the same home with animals", "SHE CALLED FOR A HALT OF GROWING ANYTHING BUT ORGANIC FOODS AROUND THE WORLD", and "she pleaded with them to use only organic foods". That is how important to health it is to rid yourself of the living pathogens that are destroying your life's time and strength and well-being. It is also to show how important it is to eat simply grown, CLEAN organic foods. And to live this very short life, even if you live to a very healthy 100, for the pleasure of the one great Creator in Heaven.

This life lasts only so long. Scripture calls it a vapor. The flesh, even though every well taken care of, does not last long! The only thing you can possibly take with you out of this life is the hope and promise of eternal life by having the Spirit of the Creator in you BEFORE you pass from this life. I urge you with every loving thought toward you to seek YOUR Creator through His Word and prayer on this with haste.

The end of this world as we know it right now is approaching fast. All indicators on every level point to it. The TRUE new world order will come after every eye sees Messiah return in the clouds just as He left this earth about 2,000 years ago. It is worth suffering for. It is worth striving for. It is worth waiting for. It is worth enduring for. Hope to see you there!

CHAPTER 75

ABOUT THE AUTHOR AND CONTACT INFORMATION

Lucinda Robinson is an herbalist since 1973 from Hickory, North Carolina, USA. She is a Messianic/Nazarene Israelite/Torah believer. She was called by the Father in heaven in 1967 and gave her life to Him in faith and obedience in June of 1970. She is married to David and has 8 grown children and 12 grandchildren. She attended Cornell University where she studied child development, nutrition, consumer advocacy, and communications. She home birthed 7 of her children and homeschooled all 8 children for a total 14 years. She loves to study nutrition, herbal and natural cures for disease, the use of essential oils for healing, the history of the paganization and heathenization of the church, the true role of women from a Scriptural perspective, home industries, Scriptural archeology, the 4,000 plus year history of Messianic Judaism, the history of dress and dress design, organic gardening, and vegan cooking and raw food preparation.

Lucinda helps individuals in their homes or care facility to address their chronic and critical health needs as a natural health care worker as well as gives lectures and seminars on health and women's spiritual issues. She is a women's torah teacher.

She counsels by appointment at her office and by phone, Skype audio and video, e-mail, and regular mail. You may contact her by e-mail at naturalherbaltherapy@gmail.com, by phone at 1-828-514-2818 and Skype at natural.herbal.therapy, or by mail at 52 Ebb Tide Drive, Palm Coast FL 32164 USA. Website is www.naturalherbaltherapy.info. Donations and payment are made through Paypal at the above email.

Lucinda Robinson is not medical doctor and has never claimed to be a medical doctor. Every client asking for help comes with a medical doctor's diagnosis in hand before counseling can start. Lucinda does not diagnose or distribute any herbal supplements. She is an herbalist counseling clients about the well known, publicly published, and proven natural treatments that have proven over many years to be effective for certain health problems using herbs, vitamins, minerals, enzymes, probiotics, and other non-invasive physical treatments. Lucinda takes no responsibility for any effects that may come from anyone trying her suggested treatments and their results in that particular person. There are so many variable possibilities that affect health that an absolute certain outcome can not be guaranteed, especially if they are not under Natural Herbal Therapy's counseling's direct contact and supervision.

GET MY MOST RECENT BOOK

SHOT DETOX!

Made in the USA
Coppell, TX
02 March 2021